PUBLIC HEALTH EMERGENCY PREPAREDNESS

A Practical Approach for the Real World

Suzet McKinney, DrPH, MPH
CEO/Executive Director
Illinois Medical District
Chicago, Illinois

Mary Elise Papke, DrPH, MPH, MA
Senior Public Health Specialist
Joseph J. Zilber School of Public Health
University of Wisconsin–Milwaukee
Milwaukee, Wisconsin

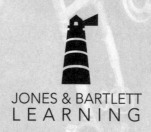

JONES & BARTLETT
LEARNING

World Headquarters
Jones & Bartlett Learning
5 Wall Street
Burlington, MA 01803
978-443-5000
info@jblearning.com
www.jblearning.com

Jones & Bartlett Learning books and products are available through most bookstores and online booksellers. To contact Jones & Bartlett Learning directly, call 800-832-0034, fax 978-443-8000, or visit our website, www.jblearning.com.

Substantial discounts on bulk quantities of Jones & Bartlett Learning publications are available to corporations, professional associations, and other qualified organizations. For details and specific discount information, contact the special sales department at Jones & Bartlett Learning via the above contact information or send an email to specialsales@jblearning.com.

Production Credits

VP, Product Management: David D. Cella
Director of Product Management: Michael Brown
Product Specialist: Carter McAlister
Production Manager: Carolyn Rogers Pershouse
Director of Vendor Management: Amy Rose
Vendor Manager: Molly Hogue
Senior Marketing Manager: Sophie Fleck Teague
Manufacturing and Inventory Control Supervisor: Amy Bacus
Composition: codeMantra U.S. LLC
Project Management: codeMantra U.S. LLC
Cover Design: Scott Moden
Rights & Media Specialist: Robert Boder
Media Development Editor: Troy Liston
Cover Image (Title Page, Part Opener, Chapter Opener): © CandyBox Images/Shutterstock
Printing and Binding: LSC Communications
Cover Printing: LSC Communications

Library of Congress Cataloging-in-Publication Data
Names: McKinney, Suzet, author. | Papke, Mary Elise, author.
Title: Public health emergency preparedness: a practical approach for the real world / Suzet McKinney, Mary Elise Papke.
Description: Burlington, Massachusetts: Jones & Bartlett Learning, [2019] | Includes bibliographical references and index.
Identifiers: LCCN 2018000272 | ISBN 9781284069259 (paperback: alk. paper)
Subjects: | MESH: Civil Defense | Emergencies | Emergency Medical Services
Classification: LCC RC451.4.D57 | NLM WA 295 | DDC 362.2/04251—dc23
LC record available at https://lccn.loc.gov/2018000272

6048

Printed in the United States of America
22 21 20 19 18   10 9 8 7 6 5 4 3 2

To Joia, You are the reason I live, breathe, and soar. My hope is that for you, I am a living example of what can be if you just believe. Grab hold of your dreams, Little One, and soar!

To David, whose support and love have been the constant in all our years together.

Contents

Preface

When we set out to write this text, our goal was very simple. We wanted to capture the experiences we have had in the field and with curriculum development in public health emergency preparedness. As public health practitioners and leaders, we know the importance of building relationships, thinking about the context of different situations, and employing strategy and a systems approach to managing complex problems. As developers of curriculum, we appreciate the challenge of synthesizing a wealth of material to stimulate learning and provoke reflection about emergency preparedness. Drawing on our experiences of practicing public health emergency preparedness and developing graduate-level certificate courses, we hope with this text to present ideas and concepts that you can translate into practice. When it comes to implementing strategies and solutions during emergencies and disasters, your practice is what is going to get you to the other side of the disaster, hopefully in a way in which illness and injury resulting from the disaster are minimized. That is the reason this text focuses on practical applications.

This text is organized into five parts. Part I, the introduction, includes the first chapter that defines public health emergency preparedness and invites readers to consider the role of public health in prevention, preparedness, response, and recovery. Chapter 2 addresses the legal issues in public health emergency preparedness. Knowledge of statutory and legal powers is invaluable for leaders charged with building and maintaining relationships, planning response actions, and seeing those actions through. It is the legal framework that guides preparedness and response strategies and tactics; understanding the legal powers afforded to the three levels of government is necessary to fully grasp when and where these legal powers will impact planning and response.

Part II of the text shifts to specific hazards and threats. Chapter 3 focuses on chemical, biological, radiological, nuclear, and explosives threats, also known as CBRNE. These threats, most commonly associated with terrorism, primarily represent high-impact, but low-probability events. Nonetheless, effective preparedness and response capability for these threats are critical. The anthrax attacks of 2001, the Boston Marathon bombing, and transportation system attacks across the globe are all stark reminders of the degree of devastation imparted among communities and economies when these malicious acts occur. Chapter 4 covers natural disasters, from hurricanes to earthquakes to floods, as well as unintentional emergencies. Each disaster requires emphasis on particular aspects of the recovery, with related environmental and infrastructure implications. Train derailments and foodborne outbreaks also entail particular responses. With an all-hazards approach to preparedness planning, jurisdictions should have key relationships in place and access to resources to facilitate ethical and coordinated responses. In all instances, mental health considerations for first responders and residents alike are important to ensure that people can restore their lives as quickly as possible. Chapter 5 is concerned with pandemic influenza. In the United States, large numbers of people succumb to seasonal flu each year. The potential for the introduction of new, novel strains of flu into our society poses specific risks that must be carefully planned for and mitigated. In this chapter, we aim to help practitioners understand how flu viruses reach pandemic level and the extreme societal impacts that pandemics can have. Chapter 6 concludes this part of the text with a discussion of emerging and reemerging infectious diseases and surveillance. The ease of global travel increases the likelihood that viruses and diseases once associated with remote, exotic locations can now be introduced in the United States. As we saw with the Ebola and Zika outbreaks in 2014 and 2015, respectively, emerging and reemerging infectious diseases can quickly overwhelm our emergency response and healthcare systems. Our unfamiliarity with these threats and limited understanding of the science behind them force us to quickly shift course to build specific capacity that stresses both our systems and economies (e.g., Ebola treatment centers).

Part III of the text turns attention to the preparedness cycle. In Chapter 7, readers learn about hazard assessment and planning, and Chapter 8 discusses training, exercising, and evaluation. What is so important about this part of the text is the presentation of the framework that is at the heart of preparedness work. There is a wealth of federal resources on these topics, from Federal Emergency Management Agency online courses to the materials from the Homeland Security Exercise and Evaluation Program (HSEEP).

In Part IV, incident management is presented beginning with multiagency coordination in Chapter 9. It is often stated that "an emergency is not the time to distribute business cards." Relationship building and understanding of partners are critical during emergency response and having those relationships in place contributes to effective incident management when it matters most. Chapter 10 discusses the psychosocial impacts of disasters, underscoring the importance of mental health resources as part of response and recovery efforts. Chapter 11 is about crisis and emergency risk communication. Communication is often the single failure point in many disaster responses. Our goal in this chapter is to give the reader an understanding of the basic strategies associated with crisis and risk communication, as well as how communication with the public is vital to the success of both the emergency response and the community's ability to quickly recover. Medical countermeasures are the topic in Chapter 12. Much planning goes into communities' creation of points of dispensing, with the attendant issues related to the logistics of meeting the needs of many people in a short time frame, an undertaking that is outside of the realm of expertise of public health. Part IV concludes with Chapter 13, which focuses on medical surge. In emergency situations, healthcare facilities need to be able to adequately provide medical evaluation and care. This chapter discusses the challenges faced by public health and the healthcare system to develop and maintain the capability to provide medical care during and after emergencies and disasters.

Finally, Chapter 14 in Part V, the conclusion, offers some thoughts on leadership. Specifically, meta-leadership is offered as a framework for approaching preparedness planning, response, and recovery. As threats become increasingly more severe and impactful, we will constantly be challenged with the need to employ more creative mechanisms for mitigating their effects. Leaders need to plan, be flexible, and remain calm in the face of disaster. We use this chapter to help practitioners understand the important role of leadership in emergency response and what distinguishes leaders from managers, and the visioning work that must take place to become a "prepared leader."

There is much to learn about this ever-changing field. As the recovery continues from Hurricanes Harvey, Irma, and Maria, we are struck by the staggering amount of work to be done to clean up and restore lives in devastated communities across eastern Texas, Florida, Puerto Rico, and the Virgin Islands. At the same time, there are countless stories of resilience in the face of extreme rain, flooding, and winds. Public and private entities are working together to bring in needed supplies, begin rebuilding, and restore services. Ever present are the social, economic, and political factors that both shape our response and influence our perceptions of responses at the local, state, and federal levels. Analysis of and reflection on each event are important to ensure that critical decisions that protect marginalized communities, restore essential services, and support our fellow citizens, especially the most vulnerable among us, can be made the next time.

We hope that we have provided you with simple, yet thought-provoking approaches to the various challenges you will face as a practitioner in this field. We encourage you to use it to expand your knowledge, challenge your thinking, and act creatively and with compassion in your approach to emergencies and disaster response.

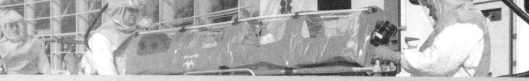

Acknowledgments

We would like to thank our longtime mentor and advisor, Dr. Bernard "Barney" Turnock, for his support and encouragement. He served as the chair of both of our doctoral dissertation committees, and was instrumental in urging us on and insisting that we always strive for excellence in the practice of public health. Barney admonished us when he felt like we needed a good kick in the pants, and pushed us when we both wanted to give up. It was Barney who introduced us to Jones & Bartlett Learning and our no-holds-barred, hard-driving publisher, Mike Brown. To Mike and our editorial team at Jones & Bartlett Learning, Carter McAlister, Lindsay Sousa, and Merideth Tumasz, your patience and understanding are more appreciated than you know. Thank you for believing in this project, even when we were not sure ourselves.

Dr. McKinney thanks her husband and daughter for all their love, support, and encouragement, not just through the writing of this book, but for everything. You are the reason why I do the work that I do. I love you, and hope that I make you proud, always.

Dr. McKinney also wishes to thank Virginia Papke, the BEST research assistant there is! Finally, Dr. McKinney wishes to acknowledge her time spent at the Chicago Department of Public Health, where she worked for nearly 14 years developing her knowledge and expertise in public health emergency preparedness and response. To Dr. Terry Mason, thank you for believing that I could lead such a large and complex operation and for demanding that I do so.

Dr. Papke would like to acknowledge Suzet for inviting her to join her as coauthor. We began our collaboration developing the curriculum for a graduate preparedness certificate and continued our dialogue about public health emergency preparedness in this book. It has been a stimulating and rewarding experience!

Dr. Papke also thanks her daughter, Virginia Papke, whose research and technical support were critical to the success of this book. She was always willing to jump into whatever task we had, no matter how picky or wide open.

Dr. Papke thanks her colleagues on the sixth floor in the UIC MidAmerica Center for Public Health Practice for introducing her to the world of public health emergency preparedness and for providing her with a wonderfully supportive work environment.

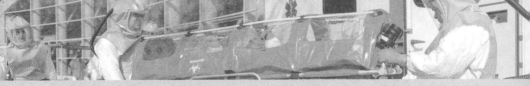

About the Authors

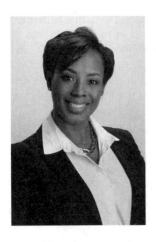

Dr. Suzet M. McKinney currently serves as Chief Executive Officer/Executive Director of the Illinois Medical District. The Illinois Medical District (IMD), a 24/7/365 environment that includes 560 acres of hospitals, medical research facilities, labs, a biotech business incubator, universities, raw land development areas, and more than 40 healthcare-related facilities, is one of the largest urban medical districts in the United States. Dr. McKinney is the former Deputy Commissioner of the Bureau of Public Health Preparedness and Emergency Response at the Chicago Department of Public Health, where she oversaw the emergency preparedness efforts for the department and coordinated those efforts within the larger spectrum of the City of Chicago's Public Safety activities. Dr. McKinney previously served as the Senior Advisor for Public Health and Preparedness at the Tauri Group, where she provided strategic and analytical consulting services to the U.S. Department of Homeland Security's BioWatch Program. Her work at the Department of Homeland Security included providing creative, responsive, and operationally based problem-solving for public health, emergency management, and homeland security issues, specifically chemical and biological early detection systems and the implementation of those systems at the state and local levels.

Dr. McKinney has earned a reputation as an experienced, knowledgeable public health official with exceptional communication skills. She has served as an on-camera media expert on emergency issues including biological and chemical threats, natural disasters, pandemic influenza, and climate-related emergencies. A sought-after expert in her field, she has also provided support to the U.S. Department of Defense's Defense Threat Reduction Agency, offering subject matter expertise in biological terrorism preparedness to international partners.

In academia, Dr. McKinney serves as an instructor in the Division of Translational Policy and Leadership Development at Harvard University's T.H. Chan School of Public Health. She also serves as a mentor for the Biomedical Sciences Careers Project at Harvard University. Additionally, Dr. McKinney holds an appointment as Adjunct Assistant Professor of Environmental and Occupational Health Sciences at the University of Illinois at Chicago School of Public Health.

Dr. McKinney holds her doctorate degree from the University of Illinois at Chicago School of Public Health, with a focus on preparedness planning, leadership, and workforce development. She received her Bachelor of Arts in Biology from Brandeis University (Waltham, Massachusetts), where she was also a Howard Hughes Medical Institute Fellow. She received her Master of Public Health degree in Health Care Administration and certificates in Managed Care and Health Care Administration from Benedictine University (Lisle, Illinois).

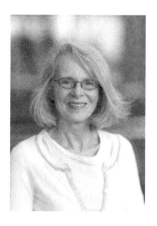

Dr. Mary Elise Papke is the Director of Accreditation Assessment and Community Engagement at the University of Wisconsin–Milwaukee Joseph J. Zilber School of Public Health. The Zilber School received its initial accreditation from the Council on Education for Public Health in 2017. She is also Senior Special Lecturer for the Master of Public Health Field Experience and Capstone courses. Dr. Papke served as adjunct faculty in the fall of 2016 at the Marquette University Law School where she co-taught a seminar in law and public health. She has extensive experience in academic public health, having served as Master of Public Health Director at the Indiana University–Purdue University at Indianapolis School of Medicine, in the Department of Public Health (now the Richard M. Fairbanks School of Public Health), and as instructional designer at the University of Illinois at Chicago School of Public Health, with the former Illinois Preparedness and Emergency Response Learning Center in the Mid-America Center for Public Health Practice. In this capacity, Dr. Papke worked on projects with the Cook County Health Department and Illinois Department of Public Health.

Currently, Dr. Papke is the affiliate representative from the Wisconsin Public Health Association to the Governing Council of the American Public Health Association. In this capacity, she is also a member of the Great Lakes Public Health Coalition. She is past president of both the Wisconsin and Indiana Public Health Associations.

Dr. Papke received her doctorate in public health from the University of Illinois at Chicago School of Public Health with a focus on organizational learning in local health departments. She earned a Master of Public Health degree in Health Services Administration from the Yale University School of Public Health, the Master of Arts degree in French Literature from New York University, and a Bachelor of Arts degree from Manhattanville College.

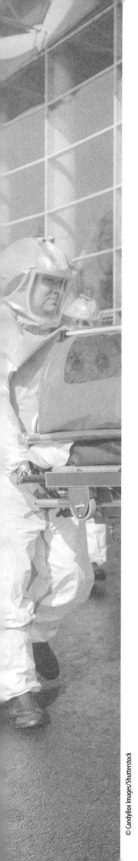

PART I

Introduction

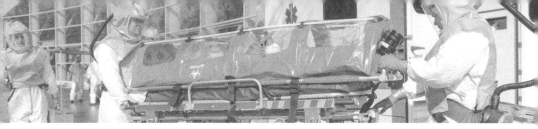

CHAPTER 1

What Is Public Health Emergency Preparedness?

LEARNING OBJECTIVES

Public health emergency preparedness is a highly specialized area of public health practice. In order to effectively appreciate the importance of public health preparedness in keeping populations healthy following a large-scale public health emergency, the basic foundations of public health practice must be placed into context with emergency and disaster situations. By the end of this chapter, readers should be able to:

- Explain the role of public health in emergency preparedness
- Describe the role of state and local governments in preparedness and response
- Describe the Incident Command System (ICS) and the importance of a centralized command structure during response operations
- Articulate the premise of the "whole community" approach to preparedness and response

▶ What Is Public Health?

In its groundbreaking report, *The Future of Public Health*, the Institute of Medicine defines public health in terms of its mission to "fulfill society's interest in assuring conditions in which people can be healthy," and the report further depicts public health's "aim to generate organized community effort to address the public interest in health by applying scientific and technical knowledge to prevent disease and promote health."[1(p7)] Unlike traditional medical care, public health employs policies and interventions to minimize disease and improve health outcomes for populations, as opposed to narrowly focusing on how to address the health of an individual. Public health is "measured in terms of improved health status, diseases prevented, scarce resources saved and improved quality of life."[2(p2)] Improvements in health due to public health scientific advancements, such as the use of vaccines and sanitation practices to prevent the spread of disease, are distinct scientific interventions. However, the public typically does not link public health's work with its achievements.

The three core functions of public health—assessment, policy development, and assurance—characterize and shape how public health practitioners approach their work. Assessment deals with the collection and analysis of health status information for communities. Policy development deals with the development of policies and the determination of appropriate interventions to address the problems in health. Finally, assurance deals with the responsibility of public health to implement strategies and interventions to promote health. Similarly, emergency preparedness as a discipline utilizes a systematic approach, the preparedness cycle, to preparing for emergencies and disasters. The steps of hazard/vulnerability assessment, planning, and mitigation/response can be likened to the three core functions of public health.

▶ What Is Emergency Preparedness?

What is public health emergency preparedness? Public health emergency preparedness is the ability to prevent, prepare for, protect against, respond to, and recover from health emergencies. Public health emergencies are emergencies whose "scale, timing, or unpredictability threaten to overwhelm routine capabilities" to provide health care.[3(pS9)] These emergencies are characterized by their high severity, inability to be managed with routine resources, and tendency to cause increased illness, injury, or death. Public health emergencies span a broad range of emergency and disaster situations, including natural hazards, acts of terrorism, and large-scale infectious disease outbreaks. We discuss the various types of emergency and disaster events more thoroughly in Chapters 4 and 5.

▶ History of Preparedness Programs/ Preparedness Funding

Public health preparedness programs in the United States started in the late 1990s. In 1999, the U.S. Centers for Disease Control and Prevention established the "Public Health Preparedness and Response for Bioterrorism Program." This program was narrowly focused on preparing for a biological terrorism attack on the United States. At that time, the threat was considered to be remote, and as such, little funding was allocated to public health for this effort. Public health agencies across the United States conducted planning for a response to a bioterrorism attack; however, the sense of urgency in this preparation was limited, as bioterrorism was thought to be a high-impact, but low-probability threat. The World Trade Center attacks in New York City on September 11, 2001 (9/11), and the subsequent anthrax attacks on the United States in October 2001 changed this thinking. With these two events came the sharp realization that the United States could not properly respond to a large-scale bioterrorism attack on the country. This was due in large part to the severely depleted infrastructure of the U.S. public health system. As a result, Congress appropriated $1 billion to public health to build the public health infrastructure in a manner that would strengthen the country's ability to respond to a bioterrorism attack. **FIGURES 1-1A** and **1-1B** illustrate funding levels since the beginning of the Public Health Emergency Preparedness (PHEP) Cooperative Agreement and the Hospital Preparedness Program Cooperative Agreement funding. Funding was allocated to 62 public health awardees, including the state health departments in all 50 states, 8 territories, and 4 directly funded cities. These directly funded cities—Chicago, New York City, Los Angeles County, and the District of Columbia—were considered to have the highest risk of a terrorist attack and thus the need to be funded separately from their states.

Public Health Emergency Preparedness (PHEP) cooperative agreement funding[1]

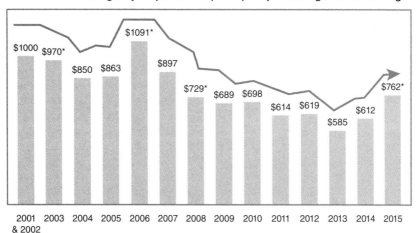

[1]Annual totals include PHEP Base Funding plus one or more of the following: Cities Readiness Initiative, Chemical Laboratory Capacity, Early Warning Infection Disease Surveillance (EWIDS), Real-Time Disease Detection, Risk Funding, Smallpox, Pandemic Influenza Supplement - Phase I, Pandemic Influenza Supplement - Phase II, Pandemic Influenza Supplement - Phase III and Ebola Supplemental Funding.

*Asterisk denotes increase in PHEP awards due to emergency supplemental funding (2003 for smallpox; 2006, 2007, and 2008 for pandemic influenza; and 2015 for Ebola). The FY2008 total includes $24 million for pandemic influenza preparedness projects that were from a different, competitive funding opportunity announcement.

FIGURE 1-1A PHEP Cooperative Agreement funding history

Data from Centers for Disease Control and Prevention. Office of Public Health Preparedness and Response.

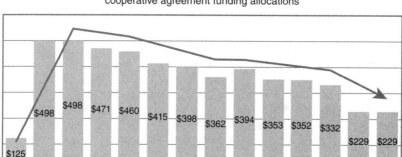

FIGURE 1-1B HPP Cooperative Agreement funding

Data from U.S. Department of Health and Human Services. Office of the Assistant Secretary for Preparedness and Response.

The initial work of the expansion of bioterrorism programs in the United States focused the role of public health as being a critical leader in the country's response to a terrorist attack.[4] This work focused on seven areas: preparedness planning and readiness assessment (focus area A), surveillance and epidemiology capacity (focus area B), laboratory capacity—biological agents (focus area C), laboratory capacity—chemical agents (focus area D), health alert networks/communications and information technology (focus area E), risk communication and health information dissemination (focus area F), and education and training (focus area G). Jurisdictions conducted planning activities around these focus areas, as well as cross-cutting areas that were integrated with hospital preparedness benchmarks and requirements funded by the Health Resources and Services Administration.[5] NOTE: The HPP Cooperative Agreement was moved from HRSA to the Office of the Assistant Secretary for Preparedness and Response when this office was created in 2006 by the Pandemic and All-Hazards Preparedness Act, or PAHPA.

In the years after 9/11, public health has used preparedness funding to plan and prepare for the aftereffects of a bioterrorism attack. However, since that time, preparedness programs have evolved from the original focus on bioterrorism attacks. This evolution of focus is not to negate the possibility of a biological, chemical, or other form of terrorist activity; however, the emergence of large-scale infectious disease outbreaks and the increase in catastrophic natural disasters have led public health to an "all-hazards" approach to public health preparedness. There is greater recognition and understanding now that most emergencies are not acts of terrorism, but are most likely natural disasters such as floods, hurricanes, and tornados, or large-scale infectious diseases such as pandemic influenza, or severe respiratory infections and zoonotic diseases, such as Ebola. Public health has also become an integral component of the emergency response community, as an accepted first responder. Public health's role as a first responder was initiated by the 9/11 attacks and subsequent anthrax attacks in 2001. This new role represented a culture shift for both public health and traditional first responders. For public health professionals, integration into the first responder community has been a big learning curve. One such example is the ICS and the National Incident Management System (NIMS) and the new language that public health first responders had to learn in order to communicate with other first responders when working alongside them during response operations.

▶ The Incident Command System and the National Incident Management System

The ICS is an organizational structure designed to assure an organized, coordinated, rapid, and seamless response to an emergency. The ICS was created in the early 1970s by the National Fire Service as a means of managing the response to forest fires in California. Developed to manage emergencies of various sizes and scopes, the ICS provides a mechanism for managing personnel, facilities, equipment, and communications.[6] Additionally, the ICS provides a common language among multiple responders, clearly identifies the chain of command and reporting structure, is cost-effective and flexible to meet the needs of emergencies of various scales, and can be used for routine operations as well as emergencies.

Today, the ICS is used by the Federal Emergency Management Agency (FEMA) and emergency management agencies across the country. Hospitals and healthcare systems have also adopted a form of ICS that is modified to suit their needs. The Hospital Incident Command System (HICS) applies the structure of ICS within hospitals and healthcare systems to enhance preparedness and response capability within healthcare institutions.[7] Like the application of ICS to public health, this system proved to be a learning curve for healthcare professionals, although it has increased coordination not only within the healthcare sector but also among officials in local and state governments.

In public health, we use what many have termed the Public Health Incident Command System (PHICS). The PHICS has become critically important to public health. Since the recognition of public health as a first responder, public health has struggled with this new role. Public health officials and other first responders have been challenged to work in concert, in both planning and response to emergencies.[8] This increased coordination, the need to forge new partnerships, and the need to integrate with other public safety partners, represented a struggle for public health, but public health responders have found that the system provides everyone with a common language, which facilitates coordination and communication across disciplines.

The traditional ICS structure includes the incident commander and four functional sections: planning, logistics, operations, and finance/administration. Surveillance and epidemiologic response efforts are usually included as a fifth functional section, or as a component of the operations section. This is important in public health response efforts because surveillance drives public health response, particularly where disease occurrence is the identified threat. Surveillance enables public health to apply the science of epidemiology to determine the causative agent of disease and track the disease trends to limit the spread (**FIGURE 1-2**).

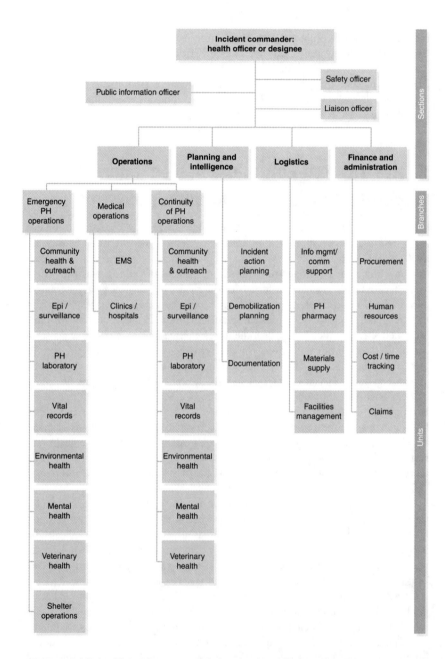

FIGURE 1-2 Public health incident command chart (epi/surveillance within operations section)

Reproduced from Rottman S, Shoaf K, Dorian A. Writing a Disaster Plan: A Guide for Health Departments. July 2005; First edition. Available at: www.ualbanycphp.org/pinata/phics/guide/fig02.cfm Accessed: January 10, 2015.

▶ Presidential Policy Directive-8 (PPD-8) and the Whole Community Approach to Preparedness

Preparedness is a shared responsibility, and as such, preparedness activities should be undertaken with a "whole community" approach.[9] While many preparedness efforts will be coordinated and led by government agencies, those agencies should engage individuals, communities, private-sector businesses, hospitals, and healthcare systems in planning and other preparedness activities. These critical stakeholders can bring great value during the planning process, but can also assist government officials during an emergency response by fostering community and institutional recovery following a disaster. Disasters that are significantly large in their scale and scope may require response assistance from state and federal government partners, as all levels of government have a role in emergency response. However, all emergencies are inherently local first. This means that local governments must be prepared to initiate emergency responses and have the capability to maintain those responses for a minimal amount of time, generally 72 hours. Engagement of the whole community can help ensure a more comprehensive, robust response. The concept of this shared responsibility is further strengthened by PPD-8. Enacted in March 2011 by President Barack Obama, PPD-8 calls for a systematic approach to preparedness for all-hazards threats and disasters. Based on the tenet that all persons possess abilities that can contribute to the nation's security, PPD-8 further calls upon the federal government to develop a national preparedness goal and core capabilities to guide activities and ensure a system-wide approach to preparedness.[10]

▶ Role of State and Local Governments in Preparedness and Response

More than the management of a single emergency or disaster event, emergency preparedness is a process. It is the process of assessing jurisdictional hazards and vulnerabilities to determine which threats are most likely to occur within a given area (community, jurisdiction, city, county, region, state). Once the most likely hazards have been identified, operational plans are developed to describe actions that will be undertaken to mitigate the hazards identified during the assessment. Preparedness plans should employ an "all-hazards" approach, with specific details given to the most likely threats, as identified by the hazard vulnerability assessment. Plans need to be scalable, flexible, and operationally sound in order to be viable during a response. Preparedness plans should be living, breathing documents. This means no good plan is ever final. Instead, the plan is reviewed with regularity, generally on an annual basis.

Those with responsibilities within the plan need to be trained to ensure achievement of the necessary competencies to execute the plan. Drills and exercises should be conducted to test the viability of the plan, and finally, the strengths and weaknesses are analyzed as a means of evaluating the plan. This is also the point at which improvement actions are identified and documented. This entire process of hazard identification, planning, training, exercising, and evaluation is frequently referred to as the preparedness cycle (see **FIGURE 1-3**).[11]

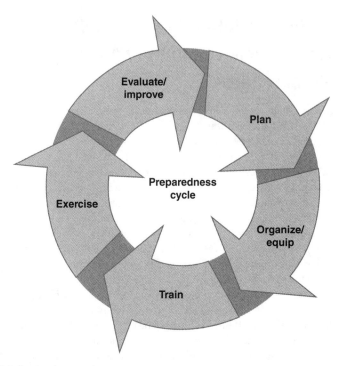

FIGURE 1-3 Preparedness cycle

Reproduced from Federal Emergency Management Agency. Preparedness Cycle. Available at: www.fema.gov/media-library/assets/images/114295#. Accessed August 29, 2017.

As previously stated, all events are inherently local and local jurisdictions must ensure they have the capability to properly respond to emergency events, and sustain themselves for minimally 72 hours. This is not to say that assistance will not be available prior to 72 hours; however, this is the generally accepted timeframe for self-sustainment. Once local resources have become exhausted, localities should request assistance from state level entities. State governments are expected to provide needed assistance to localities up until the state resources are overwhelmed or exhausted. At this point in the response, state governments can request further assistance from the federal government.

Prior to an event, state and local governments can augment their access to resources by entering into mutual aid agreements with neighboring jurisdictions or other partners. Provided the neighboring jurisdiction or partner is not affected by the same disaster, it is reasonably expected that aid will be provided. This is one strategy state and local governments can employ to achieve a longer period of self-sustainment before additional assistance is requested from the state or federal government. Mutual aid agreements are discussed further in Chapter 13.

▶ What Is the Role of Public Health in Emergency Preparedness?

Public health's role in emergency preparedness is to plan the effective strategies to minimize morbidity and mortality following an emergency or disaster. As a starting point, public health is responsible for participation in the hazard vulnerability assessment of the community or jurisdiction. In the identification of threats and hazards, public health officials should be evaluating the expected consequences of the hazard event, specifically looking to identify health and medical consequences that are likely to occur. Once the relevant threats and hazards, along with their consequences, are identified, work moves to the planning phase. In this phase, public health is responsible for identifying actions, strategies, systems, and resources that are necessary to minimize morbidity and mortality should the hazard or threat occur. Potential actions that public health officials might identify include the initiation of surveillance and epidemiological investigations to determine the source and spread of the disease or other hazard as well as the determination of potential treatment options, including laboratory testing, medical countermeasures, and the appropriateness of quarantine and isolation measures or other nonpharmaceutical interventions. Strategies to limit the spread of disease and illness frequently involve efforts to isolate the disease and implement targeted measures aimed at mitigating the threat.

Often in emergency preparedness, public health officials become overwhelmed when planning for particularly complex hazards and threats. This sense of "overwhelmness" is spurred by a misperception that public health is responsible for all aspects of threat mitigation. In fact, public health is not responsible for all aspects of emergency response, but is, however, responsible for engaging the appropriate stakeholders and partners who hold specific expertise that will aid in the emergency response or those who may also play a role in the response effort. Engagement of community and social service partners who can lend expertise in planning for the needs of at-risk, access, and functional needs persons is critical. Faith-based organizations hold strong trust relationships with community members and have an in-depth knowledge of the needs of the community. Thus, they are uniquely positioned to provide support and assistance not only during the planning phase but also in response.

Public health is also responsible for engagement and coordination with the healthcare system, namely, hospitals, community clinics, long-term care facilities, specialty providers, and other public health entities. Other healthcare system partners could include but are not limited to blood banks, dialysis centers, mental health providers, and home healthcare providers. Public health has a unique role in healthcare system coordination—that of coordinating collaboration among the multiple healthcare partners and ensuring that healthcare partners are equipped with supplies, equipment, and other resources that foster preparedness capability across the healthcare system. Just as no good plan is ever complete, neither is public health's role in emergency preparedness. Public health's planning and coordination role should continuously evolve, employing lessons learned from drills, exercises, and real events to validate and improve mitigation strategies, engaging new partners and refining a system's approach to emergency response.

▶ Importance of Public Health Infrastructure and Capacity Building

To effectively fulfill its role in emergency preparedness and response, public health needs to maintain a strong infrastructure. Public health infrastructure includes maintenance of core public health capabilities and relationships that can aid emergency response efforts. The most important of these core public health capabilities is surveillance and epidemiology. As the study of diseases and injuries in human populations, disease patterns, and the frequency of occurrence, epidemiology is considered to be the basic science of public health.[12] Epidemiologists conduct outbreak investigations to determine the origin of outbreaks, identify the populations at risk, and characterize the modes of disease transmission. Findings from these investigations are then used to initiate the efforts to control the outbreak and to prevent similar occurrences from happening in the future. Public health surveillance is the mechanism in which diseases and other health conditions are tracked. This too is an important core public health capability. Surveillance data can provide public health officials with important information that can be used to determine the subsets of the population who are affected by a particular condition. Public health surveillance and epidemiological investigation are cornerstones in public health responses to emergencies. Public health must have the ability to maintain and support routine surveillance and investigation processes and systems such that these systems can expand in response to incidents of public health significance.

While epidemiology and surveillance provide critical data and information that fuel public health response, there are many other capabilities that public health agencies must develop in order to ensure full capacity to respond to emergency events. The CDC's Public Health Preparedness Capabilities: National Standards for State and Local Planning are discussed in Chapter 7. These capabilities describe the trainings, skills, equipment and other resources that public health must have, or have access to, in order to properly respond to an emergency or disaster.

Other important aspects of public health infrastructure include human resource and financial management systems. These systems are needed in emergency response in order to maintain employee records, track employee time, and appropriately compensate employees for time worked. Inventory management and communication systems are also necessary to ensure appropriate tracking of equipment, supplies, and staff.

▶ Federal Response Structure: National Response Plan (NRP), National Response Framework (NRF)

The NRP was developed in December 2004 and established a single, comprehensive framework for the management of domestic incidents.[13] More specifically, the NRP established a progressive approach to emergency response, dictating that emergency response begin locally, flow to the state government once local resources are exhausted, and then flow to the federal government at the point that state resources become overwhelmed or are exhausted. The NRP also established multiple coordinating structures, which were designed to effectively guide and coordinate site-specific incident management activities, as well as coordination for management of disasters with national significance.

In 2008, the NRP was replaced by the NRF, which was a more comprehensive guidance that incorporated lessons learned from several events of national significance, most notably Hurricane Katrina.[14]

The NRF builds on the NIMS and strives to guide national response to emergencies and improve coordination among all response partners. The NRF aligns key roles and responsibilities to foster response partnerships at all levels of government with nongovernmental organizations and the private sector. In doing so, the NRF further promotes the "whole community" approach to preparedness and response, as established by PPD-8, and thus should be used by the whole community for emergency preparedness and response. The priorities of the NRF are to "save lives, protect property and the environment, stabilize the incident and provide for basic human needs."[15(9pg i)] To meet these priorities, the NRF establishes a response vision through five key principles:

1. **Engaged partnership**: All levels of government and the whole community must develop shared response goals and align capabilities to ensure no one entity is overwhelmed in times of crisis.
2. **Tiered response**: Incidents must be managed at the lowest possible jurisdictional level (local) and supported by additional capabilities when needed.
3. **Scalable, flexible, adaptable operational capabilities**: As incidents change in size, scope, and complexity, the response must adapt to meet these changing requirements.
4. **Unity in response through unified command**: Respect the chain of command of participating organizations and ensure seamless coordination across jurisdictions in support of common objectives.
5. **Readiness to act**: Ensure the best response possible that is grounded in a clear understanding of potential risks and decisive actions.

The NRF is composed of multiple components that can be used together or independently, based on the nature, scope, and scale of the emergency. Those components include the base document, Emergency Support Function (ESF) Annexes, Support Annexes, and Incident Annexes (**FIGURE 1-4**).

As indicated in the guidance document, the annexes provide detailed information to assist with the implementation of the NRF. ESF Annexes describe the federal coordinating structures that group resources and capabilities into functional areas that are most frequently needed in a national response. Support Annexes describe the essential

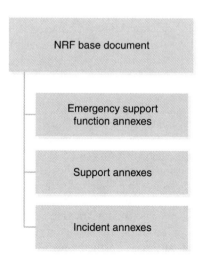

FIGURE 1-4 Structure of the NRF

Data from FEMA. National Response Framework. Available at: www.fema.gov/media-library-data/20130726-1914-25045-1246/final_national_response_framework_20130501.pdf. Accessed January 27, 2015.

supporting processes and considerations that are most common to the majority of incidents. Incident Annexes describe the unique response aspects of incident categories.

▶ The Public Health Workforce and Development of Preparedness Competencies and Association of Schools and Programs of Public Health Core Competencies

Ensuring the public health workforce develops and maintains the appropriate skills, knowledge, and competencies for responding to emergency events is a critical component of the development of emergency preparedness capability. For many years, specific preparedness competency remained a mystery. Early iterations of preparedness competency were developed by staff at the Columbia University School of Nursing, Center for Health Policy. The Pandemic and All-Hazards Preparedness Act called for a comprehensive, competency-based training program that is responsive to the needs of state, local, and tribal public health organizations and emphasizes public health security capabilities. In response to the call for the development of a comprehensive competency framework for educational programs in public health emergency preparedness, the Association of Schools and Programs of Public Health developed the Master's Preparedness & Response Model.[16] This model was designed for use by graduate level educational programs to ensure students obtain the necessary knowledge, skills and attitudes associated with public health emergency preparedness and response. Under this model, students should gain competency in roles and relationships, communication and information management, planning and improvement, assessment and incident management. The model's framework is based on a series of tenets that are all designed to build competency in future generations of the public health workforce with particular expertise in preparedness and response.

▶ Conclusion

Public health emergency preparedness is the ability to prevent, prepare for, protect against, respond to, and recover from health emergencies. As the scope, size, and scale of public health emergencies continue to increase, it is more and more important for public health to maintain the ability to respond to threats and hazards that impact the public's health. While public health preparedness programs date back to the late 1990s, those early programs were narrowly focused. These programs became top of mind for many Americans following the 2001 anthrax attacks in New York City, Florida, and Washington, DC, yet they remained narrowly focused on biological threats. With the increased occurrence of different types of threats, the focus of preparedness programs has now adjusted to include all-hazards emergencies.

The NIMS and the ICS provide responders with a coordinated framework within which to operate during emergency response efforts. While difficult for public health workers to grasp initially, these concepts are now widely accepted and used as the standard framework for managing disasters of all sizes, with participation by multiple agencies and jurisdictions.

Discussion Questions

1. What is public health emergency preparedness?
2. Describe the incidents that led to the creation and/or expansion of public health emergency preparedness programs in the United States.
3. What is the role of state and local governments in preparedness and response? What is meant by the phrase "whole community approach to preparedness"?
4. What is the ICS, and why is it important to preparedness and response?

References

1. Institute of Medicine. *The Future of Public Health.* Washington, DC: National Academy Press; 1988.
2. Turnock B. *Public Health: What It Is and How It Works.* 5th ed. Burlington, MA: Jones & Bartlett Learning; 2012.
3. Nelson C, Lurie N, Wasserman J, Zakowski S. Conceptualizing and defining public health emergency preparedness. *Am J Public Health.* 2007;97(S1):S9–S11.
4. Centers for Disease Control and Prevention. Biological and chemical terrorism: strategic plan for preparedness and response. *MMWR.* 2000;49(no. RR04):1–14. Available at http://www.cdc.gov/mmwr/preview/mmwrhtml/rr4904a1.htm.
5. Centers for Disease Control and Prevention. Continuation guidance for cooperative agreement on public health preparedness and response for bioterrorism—budget year five program announcement, June 14, 2004. Available at http://www.cdc.gov/phpr/documents/coopagreement-archive/FY2004/guidance_intro.pdf. Accessed January 5, 2015.
6. U.S. Department of the Interior, National Park Service. Fire and aviation management, incident command system. Available at https://www.nps.gov/fire/wildland-fire/learning-center/fire-in-depth/incident-command-system.cfm. Accessed January 10, 2015.
7. Hospital Incident Command System. The Center for HICS Education and Training. Available at http://hicscenter.org/SitePages/Mission.aspx. Accessed January 10, 2015.
8. Werner D, Wright K, Thomas M, Edgar M. An innovation in partnership among first responders and public health: bridging the gap. *Public Health Rep.* 2005;120(S1):64–68. Available at http://www.ncbi.nlm.nih.gov/pmc/articles/PMC2569990/pdf/phr120s10064.pdf.
9. FEMA. A whole community approach to emergency management: principles, themes, and pathways for action. December 2011. Available at http://www.fema.gov/media-library-data/20130726-1813-25045-0649/whole_community_dec2011__2_.pdf. Accessed January 25, 2015.
10. Department of Homeland Security. Presidential policy directive/PPD-8: national preparedness. Available at http://www.dhs.gov/presidential-policy-directive-8-national-preparedness. Last Published January 15, 2014. Accessed January 25, 2015.
11. FEMA. National preparedness cycle. Available at https://www.fema.gov/national-preparedness-cycle. Last Updated July 24, 2014. Accessed January 27, 2015.
12. Dworkin M. *Cases in Field Epidemiology: A Global Perspective.* 1st ed. Burlington, MA: Jones & Bartlett Learning; 2011.
13. FEMA. National response plan. Available at http://www.dhs.gov/xlibrary/assets/NRP_Brochure.pdf. Accessed January 27, 2015.
14. FEMA. National response framework. Available at https://www.fema.gov/national-response-framework. Accessed January 27, 2015.

15. FEMA. National response framework. Available at https://www.fema.gov/media-library
    -data/20130726-1914-25045-1246/final_national_response_framework_20130501.pdf.
    Accessed January 27, 2015.
16. Association of Schools & Programs of Public Health. Public health preparedness & response
    model. Available at https://www.aspph.org/teach-research/models/public-health-preparedness
    -response/. Accessed December 11, 2017.

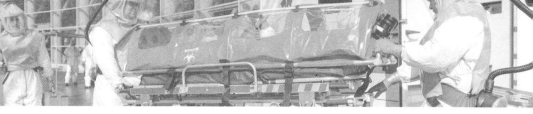

CHAPTER 2

Legal Issues in Public Health Emergency Preparedness

LEARNING OBJECTIVES

A number of policies govern federal, state, and local roles in emergency preparedness and response. Some policies determine how funding will be directed to disaster-stricken jurisdictions. Others define processes, physical assistance, and authority. Many types of federal policies guide preparedness and response activities, and it is important to understand the differences between these policies. By the end of this chapter, readers should be able to:

- Identify the key legislation that shapes public health emergency preparedness
- Explain the relationships among the local, state, and federal levels of government regarding the legal dimensions of public health emergency preparedness
- Assess the policy implications of the legal framework for public health emergency preparedness

▶ Introduction

Most observers consider the United States an extraordinarily legalistic country. Law is something of a rudder for American social life and an important one at that. It establishes frameworks, creates formal relationships, and articulates guidelines. It prescribes and proscribes. Law is perhaps the clearest and most obvious expression of public policy.

Public health law as a whole and emergency preparedness law in particular focus on protecting the health and safety of the population. Law of this sort is so important as to constitute a major part of the public health infrastructure.[1] Statutes, regulations, and judicial decisions are crucial in emergency preparedness. These statutes, regulations, and judicial decisions related to emergency preparedness can be found at the local, state, and federal levels. The laws vary from jurisdiction to jurisdiction, and the relationships among the laws at these levels of government have evolved over time for a variety of reasons.[1(pp166–167)] As a result, there are many laws in each of the states that address public health matters and emergency preparedness specifically.

One venerable but particularly controversial variety of emergency preparedness law that illustrates the variation and the changing relationships of different laws involves isolation and quarantine. Local and state governments are empowered through the police powers as defined in state constitutions to protect the public's health and safety. Isolating and quarantining those with communicable diseases in specified circumstances is one way to safeguard the public's health and safety. State statutes specify a list of diseases that must be reported to state health departments and to the Centers for Disease Control and Prevention (CDC), which maintains a national surveillance system of notifiable diseases.

The controversial nature of quarantine as a state legal power was dramatically illustrated in the states of New Jersey and Maine in 2014. A nurse named Kaci Hickox returned in October from Sierra Leone in West Africa, where she had been working with Doctors Without Borders treating patients suffering from Ebola. Upon her arrival at the Newark Airport in New Jersey, she was ordered by Governor Chris Christie to face a mandatory 21-day quarantine in New Jersey (**BOX 2-1**).

Hickox challenged the quarantine order as she had no symptoms and had tested negative for Ebola. She was then allowed to travel to Maine, where Governor Paul LePage issued a quarantine order that confined Hickox to her home. She defied that order on a bike ride near her home, and with national media focused on Maine, a judge ruled in her favor against the state. In his ruling (see **EXHIBIT 2-1**), Judge Charles LaVerdiere stated that, "The State has not met its burden at this time to prove by clear and convincing evidence that limiting Respondent's movements to the degree requested is 'necessary to protect other individuals from the dangers of infection,' however. According to the information presented to the court, Respondent currently does not show any symptoms of Ebola and is therefore *not* infectious."[2] The judge's ruling confirms the fine line between safeguarding individual rights and protecting the health of the public.[3]

The federal government is also legally authorized to use isolation and quarantine. This would be most likely if someone with a communicable disease crossed state lines or entered the United States from an international destination. In 2007, the federal government isolated Andrew Speaks in Atlanta after he had been diagnosed with a dangerous form of tuberculosis that is resistant to antibiotics (XDR TB) and returned from Europe to the United States via Montreal and New York.

BOX 2-1 Challenging a State Quarantine Order

In an interview with CNN on October 26, 2014, Kaci Hickox described her feelings on being placed in quarantine at a New Jersey hospital after returning from West Africa. "This is an extreme that is really unacceptable, and I feel like my basic human rights have been violated."

Data from Crowley C. (26 October 2014). Quarantined nurse slams new policy. State of the Union with Candy Crowley. CNN Press Room.

STATE OF MAINE
AROOSTOOK, SS.

DISTRICT COURT
Location: Fort Kent
Docket No: CV-2014-36

Mary C. Mayhew, Commissioner)
State of Maine Department of Health)
and Human Services,)
                Petitioner,)   Order Pending Hearing
      v.)
Kaci Hickox,)
                Respondent.)

The State has requested that the court issue an order restricting Respondent's activities pending the final hearing on its Verified Petition for a Public Health Order. This decision has critical implications for Respondent's freedom, as guaranteed by the U.S. and Maine Constitutions, as well as the public's right to be protected from the potential severe harm posed by transmission of this devastating disease. Given the gravity of these interests, the Court yesterday entered a temporary order maintaining the status quo until a further hearing could occur this morning. It was imperative that the court take the necessary time to review in detail the parties' submissions, the arguments of counsel, and the cases cited by counsel regarding the necessity of entering an order pending the final hearing in this matter.

Maine Law authorizes a court to "make such orders as it deems *necessary to protect other individuals from the dangers of infection*" pending a hearing on a petition for a public health order. 22 M.R.S. § 811(3) (2014) (emphasis added). At this point in time, the only information that the Court has before it regarding the dangers of infection posed by Respondent, who has potentially but not definitely been exposed to the Ebola virus, derives from the Affidavit of Shiela Pinette, D.O., Director of the Maine Center for Disease Control and Prevention, together with the attachments from the U.S. Centers for Disease Control. In her affidavit, Dr. Pinette averred, *inter alia:*

> 8. Ebola Virus Disease is spread through direct contact with the blood, sweat, vomit, feces and other body fluids *of a symptomatic person.* It can also be spread through exposure to needles or other objects contaminated with the virus.
> . . .
>
> 12. Transmission of Ebloa is usually through direct contact with the blood, sweat, emesis, feces and other body secretions of an infected person, or exposure to objects (such as needles) that have been contaminated with infected secretions.
> . . .
>
> 14. *Individuals infected with Ebola Virus Disease who are not showing symptoms are not yet infectious.* Early symptoms of Ebola are non-specific and common to many other illnesses.
>
> 15. Symptoms usually include: fever, headache, joint and muscle aches, weakness, diarrhea, vomiting, stomach pain, and lack of appetite. *Ebola may be present in an individual who does not exhibit any of these symptoms, because they are not yet infectious.*

(continues)

16. The incubation period for the virus, before it can be determined that a person does not have Ebola virus, is 21 days ("the incubation period"). A person who is infected with Ebola virus can start to show symptoms of the disease (become infectious) at any point during the incubation period. A person can test negative for Ebola virus in the early part of the incubation period and later become infectious and test positive.

17. The Respondent remains at risk of being infected with Ebola, until the 21-day time period has assed. The most common time of developing symptoms is during the second week after last exposure. Respondent entered that second week starting October 28, 2014. The surest way to minimize the public health threat is direct active monitoring and additional restrictions on movement and exposure to other persons or the public until a potentially exposed person has passed the incubation period. For Respondent that period expires November 10, 2014.

18. Symptoms usually appear 8 to 10 days after exposure and 90% of cases develop symptoms within the first 14 days of exposure. So the time of greatest risk of showing symptoms and becoming infectious is within the first 14 days of the incubation period. Once someone is displaying symptoms and is actually infected with Ebola, they become increasingly infectious and extremely ill, requiring attendance for basic daily needs within a matter of a few days. There is no known cure for Ebola.

. . .

27. Respondent is asymptomatic (no fever or other symptoms consistent with Ebola), as of the last check pursuant to her direct active monitoring this morning. Therefore the guidance issued by US CDC states that she is subject to Direct Active Monitoring. Health care workers in the "some risk" category require direct active monitoring for the 21-day incubation period.

28. Direct active monitoring means the MeCDC provides direct observation at least once per day to review symptoms and monitor temperature with a second follow-up daily by phone. The purpose of direct active monitoring is to ensure that if individuals with epidemiologic risk factors become ill, they are identified as soon as possible after symptoms onset so they can be rapidly isolated and evaluated. Once a person is symptomatic they become contagious to others, and their infectiousness increases very quickly.

. . .

(10/30/2014 Aff. of Dr. Pinette, at 2-4).

Based on the information in this affidavit with attachments and arguments of counsel, the Court finds by clear and convincing evidence that an order is necessary. With regard to the contents of the order, the court finds that ordering Respondent to comply with Direct Active Monitoring and to engage in the steps outlined below is "necessary to protect other individuals from the dangers of infection." The Court is aware that Respondent has been cooperating with Direct Active Monitoring and intends to continue with her cooperation. While this Court has no reason to doubt Respondent's good intentions, it is nevertheless necessary to ensure public safety that she continue to comply with Direct Active Monitoring until a hearing can be held on the State's Petition. The State has not met its burden at this time to prove by clear and convincing evidence that limiting Respondent's movements to the degree requested is "necessary to protect other individuals from the dangers of infection," however. According to the information presented to the court, Respondent currently does not show any symptoms of Ebola and is therefore <u>not</u> infectious. Should these circumstances change at any time before the hearing on the petition—a situation that will most quickly come to light if Direct Active Monitoring is maintained—then it will become necessary to isolate Respondent from others to prevent the potential spread of this devastating disease.

For the foregoing reasons, the Court hereby ORDERS that, pending the hearing on the petition, Respondent shall:

1. Participate in and cooperate with "Direct Active Monitoring" as that term is defined by the United States Centers for Disease Control in its October 29, 2014 *Interim U.S. Guidance for Monitoring and Movement of Persons with Potential Ebola Virus Exposure* and in paragraph 28 of Dr. Pinette's October 30, 2014 affidavit.

2. Coordinate her travel with public health authorities to ensure uninterrupted Direct Active Monitoring; and

3. <u>Immediately</u> notify public health authorities and follow their directions if <u>any</u> symptom appears.

This Order is intended to and does supersede the Temporary Order entered on October 30, 2014 in this matter.

The Court pauses to make a few critical observations. First, we would not be here today unless Respondent generously, kindly and with compassion lent her skills to aid, comfort, and care for individuals stricken with a terrible disease. We need to remember as we go through this matter that we owe her and all professionals who give of themselves in this way a debt of gratitude.

Having said that, Respondent should understand that the court is fully aware of the misconceptions, misinformation, bad science and bad information being spread from shore to shore in our country with respect to Ebola. The Court is fully aware that people are acting out of fear and that this fear is not entirely rational. However, whether that fear is rational or not, it is present and it is real. Respondent's actions at this point, as a health care professional, need to demonstrate her full understanding of human nature and the real fear that exists. She should guide herself accordingly.

Further, since Respondent has waived her right to confidentiality pursuant to 22 M.R.S. § 811(6)(E), it is hereby ORDERED that all filings, orders, and hearings in this matter shall be open to the public.

This Order shall be incorporated into the docket by reference pursuant to M.R.Civ. P. 79(a).

Dated: October 31, 2014

Charles C. LaVerdiere
Chief Judge, Maine District Court

EXHIBIT 2-1 Court Decision—Mayhew v. Hickox, State of Maine; Ebola Quarantine Case, Judge Charles LaVerdiere; October 31, 2014

Data from State of Maine Judicial Branch. High Profile Cases. State of Maine Department of Health and Human Services v. Kaci Hickox. Order Pending Hearinf Available at: www.courts.maine.gov/news_reference/high_profile/hickox.shtml. Accessed December 2, 2014.

A comprehensive consideration of all the ways the police powers at the various levels of government are used to assure the public's health is beyond the scope of this book. The focus here is on key laws, regulations, and directives related to public health emergency preparedness and response. The goal is to highlight the important features of these laws, regulations, and directives while also underscoring the political, ethical, and practical reality of this legal landscape. The chapter begins with the federal policy and statutory framework, which addresses legislation and policy regulations. It then turns to disaster declarations followed by legal considerations in planning for threats and disasters. The chapter concludes with some thoughts on legal preparedness, that is, the capacity of practitioners to be competent in their respective legal frameworks and their ability to coordinate with others across jurisdictions in evolving emergency situations, in the context of public health emergency preparedness and response.

▶ Policy and Statutory Framework

The policy and statutory framework related to public health emergency preparedness and response incorporates legislation, executive orders, and presidential decision directives. Together these legal actions provide a narrative of the evolving role of the federal government's policy approaches in public health emergency preparedness and the accompanying changes in organization to carry out these policies and regulations. This narrative is, of course, shaped not only by political factors in the different presidential administrations but also by external factors, including our relationships with other nations as well as natural and man-made events with the power to realign national priorities and shift the organizational structures needed to address these priorities. This section provides a brief summary of key legislation, executive orders, and presidential decision directives.

The Cold War between the United States and Russia influenced policies and structures during the administrations of Presidents Truman, Eisenhower, and Kennedy.[4] Over the course of the three administrations, emergency preparedness evolved, becoming more closely related to national defense. Responsibility for the government's response moved from the Housing and Home Finance Administrator to the Federal Civil Defense Administrator with the passage of the Federal Civil Defense Act in 1950 (President Truman) to the Office of Defense and Civilian Mobilization (President Eisenhower) to the Office of Emergency Planning (President Kennedy).[4,5]

Federal Emergency Management Agency (FEMA)

Several hurricanes and earthquakes in the 1960s and 1970s, especially Hurricane Agnes in 1972, underscored the inadequacy of the federal government's response to major disasters.[4,5] Important legislation during this period included the National Flood Insurance Act (1968), the Flood Disaster Protection Act (1973), and the Disaster Relief Act (1974; see discussion that follows).[4-6] By the time of President Carter's administration, the nuclear accident at Three Mile Island, Pennsylvania, had occurred in 1979,[5(pp12-15)] and over 100 federal agencies had participated in response and recovery related to emergencies of all types.[6] Authority for federal response to emergencies rested then with the Federal Disaster Assistance Administration in the Department of Housing and Urban Development.[4,5]

President Carter's *Executive Order 12127* changed the structure of the federal government's organization of emergency preparedness work, if not its approach. With input from the National Governors' Association, as well as the work of commissions following Hurricane Agnes and the Three Mile Island nuclear accident, President Carter established the Federal Emergency Management Agency, known as FEMA.[4-6] Functions that had been located in the Department of Commerce, the Department of Housing and Urban Development, and in the White House were now transferred to this new agency.[7] FEMA was responsible for coordinating national efforts related to preparation, mitigation, response, and recovery for man-made and natural emergencies.[8] However, local and state governments remained responsible for local planning, response, and recovery to the extent allowed by their resources and capacity. The federal government's role was to provide assistance.

Homeland Security Act of 2002

The next major reorganization of the federal government's emergency preparedness infrastructure followed soon after the terrorist attacks on the World Trade Center and the Pentagon on September 11, 2001, as well as the anthrax letters in October of that year. The first step in this process of addressing the national government's approach to national security, in addition to emergency preparedness, was President George W. Bush's *Executive Order 13228* on October 8, 2001, which created the Office of Homeland Security and the Homeland Security Council.[9(p50)] This action was followed by the passage of the Homeland Security Act of 2002 (PL 107-296). This Act established the Department of Homeland Security (DHS), combining 22 different agencies into one. FEMA was one of the agencies brought under the new department.[10] In the wake of 9/11 and the anthrax attacks, there was immediate legislative action.

Selected Public Health Emergency Preparedness Legislation and Homeland Security Presidential Directives

Not surprisingly, the events of 9/11 shaped the national legislative agenda in ways other than organizational. Subsequent legislation addressed various issues ranging from bioterrorism to liability from claims from the use of countermeasures to pandemics. Two Homeland Security Presidential Directives (HSPDs), meanwhile, created the framework for coordination and management among the three levels of government to address both man-made and natural disaster events. Finding the most prudent way to prevent, protect, respond to, and recover from emergency events has proved challenging. Issues related to agency authority and specific community needs may not emerge until government officials and community leaders sit down to evaluate what did, or did not, happen during and after a particular event.

Public Health Security and Bioterrorism Preparedness and Response Act of 2002

The first legislation for public health preparedness, the Public Health Security and Bioterrorism Preparedness and Response Act of 2002 (PL 107-188) is notable for the speed with which the U.S. House and U.S. Senate considered and passed the bill, and the House and Senate Conference Reports were agreed to within a day of each other.[9(p68)] There was an urgency for coordination among key federal agencies as well as an approach to planning across all levels of government.

This Public Health Security Act amended Section 319 of the Public Health Service Act, "To improve the ability of the United States to prevent, prepare for, and respond to bioterrorism and other public health emergencies."[11] Title I of the Act calls for the development of a national preparedness plan, "a coordinated strategy," that should "build[ing] upon the core public health capabilities," as spelled out in Section 319A.[12] Specific goals focused on surveillance, laboratory capacity, training, medical countermeasures, and hospital preparedness (see **BOX 2-2**).

Title I also established the position of Assistant Secretary for Public Health Emergency Preparedness in the Department of Health and Human Services (DHHS). The purpose of this position was the coordination of federal agencies and the National Disaster Medical System (see discussion of National Disaster Medical System in Chapter 13) during an emergency. The Assistant Secretary was also charged with evaluating the outcomes of the National Preparedness Plan. Other titles in the Act focused on controlling biological agents and toxins (Title II) as well as protecting food, drug, and drinking water (Titles III and IV) supplies.

BOX 2-2 National Preparedness Goals of the Public Health Security and Bioterrorism Preparedness and Response Act of 2002

SEC. 2801. NATIONAL PREPAREDNESS (b) PREPAREDNESS GOALS—The plan under subsection (a) should include provisions in furtherance of the following:

1. Providing effective assistance to State and local governments in the event of bioterrorism or other public health emergency.
2. Ensuring that State and local governments have appropriate capacity to detect and respond effectively to such emergencies, including capacities for the following:
   A. Effective public health surveillance and reporting mechanisms at the State and local levels.
   B. Appropriate laboratory readiness.
   C. Properly trained and equipped emergency response, public health, and medical personnel.
   D. Health and safety protection of workers responding to such an emergency.
   E. Public health agencies that are prepared to coordinate health services (including mental health services) during and after such emergencies.
   F. Participation in communications networks that can effectively disseminate relevant information in a timely and secure manner to appropriate public and private entities and to the public.
3. Developing and maintaining medical countermeasures (such as drugs, vaccines and other biological products, medical devices, and other supplies) against biological agents and toxins that may be involved in such emergencies.
4. Ensuring coordination and minimizing duplication of Federal, State, and local planning, preparedness, and response activities, including during the investigation of a suspicious disease outbreak or other potential public health emergency.
5. Enhancing the readiness of hospitals and other healthcare facilities to respond effectively to such emergencies.

Data from Government Publishing Office. Public Health Security and Bioterrorism Preparedness and Response Act of 2002. SEC. 2801. NATIONAL PREPAREDNESS (b) PREPAREDNESS GOALS Available at: www.gpo.gov/fdsys/pkg/PLAW-107publ188 /pdf/PLAW-107publ188.pdf. Accessed: 12/7/14

Homeland Security Presidential Directives

Two important Homeland Security Presidential Directives followed not long after the Public Health Security and Bioterrorism Preparedness Act was signed in June 2002. Issued by the National Security Council, these Homeland Security Presidential Directives reflect President George Bush's policies on bioterrorism and preparedness in the wake of 9/11.[9(p52)] In Homeland Security Presidential Directive-5 (HSPD-5), released on February 28, 2003, President Bush called for the "establish[ment] of a single, comprehensive approach to domestic incident management." The intent of this policy was to "treat[s] crisis management and consequence management as a single, integrated function, rather than two separate functions."[13] HSPD-5 called for the development and implementation of a National Incident Management System (NIMS). Together with a National Response Plan, the federal government wanted to create a "consistent approach" to preparedness, response, and recovery at all levels in "one all-discipline, all-hazards plan."[13] HSPD-5 highlights several features of incident command with implications for public health practice related to terminology and language, multiagency coordination, unified command, and training, among other topics. The plan for implementing NIMS was to be ready by August 2003.

Issued on December 17, 2003, as a companion to HSPD-5, Homeland Security Presidential Directive-8 (HSPD-8) focused on efforts in the states "to build capacity to address major events, especially terrorism."[14] In addition to the development of a national preparedness goal, the policy emphasized equipment standards for interoperability among first responders and training and exercises for all workers who would be involved in prevention, response, and recovery. An important aspect of training and exercises was sharing lessons learned and best practices through an integrated national system. Best practices for citizen participation in preparedness were also to be disseminated widely in support of local and state preparedness work. Through the creation of a national preparedness goal and implementation of consistent standards across a range of activities, the federal government sought to integrate preparedness, response, and recovery initiatives into a more seamless approach.

Public Health Readiness and Emergency Preparedness (PREP) Act of 2005

The Public Health Readiness and Emergency Preparedness Act of 2005 (PREP Act; Public Law No. 109-148; 42 USC 247d-6d and 6e) focused on another aspect of preparation for a major event, that is, medical countermeasures. Under this law, anyone involved in the development, manufacture, distribution, administration, and use of a medical countermeasure for a specific disease or potentially harmful event would not be liable for any claims of injury or loss stemming from the administration and use of such a drug or antidote or device.[10] This immunity from liability was considered especially important for those cases in which a drug or vaccine might not yet be approved by the U.S. Food and Drug Administration (FDA) but was an essential part of the government's response to protect the population from a particular threat.[9(p53)] The Secretary of the DHHS must issue a declaration that presents the specific threat and countermeasure and defines the time frame, population affected, particular geographic area if any, and distribution plan for the immunity.[15] Since January 2007, there have been declarations for immunity from liability for countermeasures for radiation, smallpox, botulism, anthrax as well as several amendments to the H5N1pandemic flu, including one for H1N1 on June 15, 2009.[16] For example, Secretary of DHHS Sylvia Burwell issued a declaration under the PREP Act in

---

BOX 2-3 Responsibilities of the Assistant Secretary of Preparedness and Response

- National Disaster Medical System
- Medical Reserve Corps
- Emergency System for Advance Registration of Volunteer Health Professionals
- Hospital Preparedness Program Cooperative Agreement
- Strategic National Stockpile
- Cities Readiness Initiative

Data from Government Publishing Office. Pandemic and All-Hazards Preparedness Act of 2006. Public Law 109-417. SEC. 102. Assistant Secretary for Preparedness and Response. December 19, 2006. 120 STAT. 2834 42 USC 300-hh-10) Available at: www .gpo.gov/fdsys/pkg/PLAW-109publ417/pdf/PLAW-109publ417.pdf. Accessed: 1/4/15.

2014 for the development of an Ebola vaccine, which was amended in early 2017, and there are also declarations for Zika virus and nerve agents.[17]

Pandemic and All-Hazards Preparedness Act of 2006

The Pandemic and All-Hazards Preparedness Act of 2006 (Public Law No. 109-417; 120 STAT. 2832) addressed organizational issues as well as security infrastructure, surge capacity, and medical countermeasures.[10] This Act established that, "The Secretary of Health and Human Services shall lead all Federal public health and medical response to public health emergencies and incidents covered by the National Response Plan developed pursuant to section 502(6) of the Homeland Security Act of 2002, or any successor plan."[18] The position of Assistant Secretary for Preparedness and Response replaced the position of Assistant Secretary for Public Health Emergency Preparedness from the 2002 Public Health Security and Bioterrorism Preparedness and Response Act. **BOX 2-3** lists several of the Assistant Secretary's responsibilities, which range from countermeasures to hospital preparedness to the Cities Readiness Initiative.

The Act required states to prepare pandemic flu plans and provided grants to states for enhancing their "public health situational awareness systems for public health emergencies,"[19] as well as for workforce and health professional volunteers training. Finally, the Act also authorized creation in DHHS of the Biomedical Advanced Research and Development Authority (BARDA; PL 109-417) to promote the development of vaccines and drugs through collaboration among a range of government, private, and academic institutions. This step was consistent with the government's goal of implementing a national security plan that addressed the issue with a variety of actions.

Pets Evacuation and Transportation Standards Act of 2006

The experience during Hurricane Katrina in 2005 of pets stranded and abandoned revealed shortcomings in planning at the local and state levels before, during, and after the storm for household pets and service animals. An amendment to the 1988 Robert T. Stafford Act (see discussion of the Stafford Act later in this chapter), the Pets Evacuation and Transportation Standards Act of 2006 (PETS; Public Law No. 109-308) focused on people with pets and service animals through planning, funds, and delivery of services. The Act authorized the FEMA director to establish standards for preparedness planning at the local and state levels for people with pets and service animals. The director could designate funds for emergency shelters for

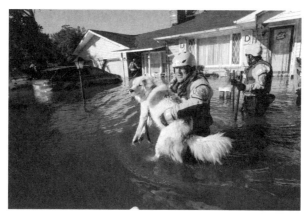

FIGURE 2-1 A dog being carried through a flooded street
Courtesy of FEMA/Jocelyn Augustino.

approved animal preparedness projects. Finally, the Act also "authorizes . . . provision of rescue, care, shelter and essential needs to individuals with household pets and service animals and to such pets and animals."[20] Images from flood-ravaged Houston, Texas, of pets being carried to safety by their owners and held wrapped in towels in shelters across the city (see **FIGURE 2-1**) illustrate the significant impact of this legislation, which had bipartisan support.[21] People knew that pets would be welcome in the shelters, which made fleeing their homes from the rising waters slightly easier.

Post-Katrina Emergency Management Reform Act of 2006

The federal government's handling of Hurricane Katrina in August 2005 prompted a reconsideration of the organization of DHS and FEMA, the first since the 2002 Homeland Security Act. The Post-Katrina Emergency Management Reform Act of 2006 was passed as part of the DHS Appropriations Act of 2007 (Public Law No. 109-295).[10] The DHS was reorganized, with some functions moving to FEMA, and FEMA's responsibilities during emergency events were increased.

Pandemic and All-Hazards Preparedness Reauthorization (PAHPRA) Act of 2013

The Pandemic and All-Hazards Preparedness Reauthorization Act (PAHPRA) of 2013 (Public Law No. 113-5) continued funding for the Hospital Preparedness Program and the Public Health Emergency Preparedness Cooperative Agreement. The Act also ensured ongoing funding for countermeasures, including drugs, vaccines, and medical equipment and supplies. Another purpose of the legislation was to promote "advanced research for and development of potential medical countermeasures" through the Bioshield Project,[22] and the FDA was given the ability to use the Emergency Use Authorization (EUA) for a given drug as a medical countermeasure before a public health emergency had been declared.[22] Finally, PAHPRA mandated that grantees' All-Hazard Preparedness plans include specific information related to children and vulnerable populations and address coordination with the local Medical Reserve Corps and Cities Readiness Initiative.[10]

Sandy Recovery Improvement Act of 2013

An amendment to Title IV of the Robert T. Stafford Act (see discussion of the Stafford Act later in this chapter), the Sandy Recovery Improvement Act of 2013 was intended to simplify disaster assistance administered by FEMA. To enhance flexibility and speed up the recovery process, eligibility criteria for individual assistance were clarified; childcare expenses were deemed allowable along with funeral, medical, and dental costs; debris removal was to be based on a cost-share program with the federal government, with incentives for local and tribal governments with specific contractors in place before the declaration of a major disaster; and FEMA could lease multifamily housing to speed up the resettlement process.[23] In addition, tribal leaders of federally recognized nations would be able to request an emergency or major disaster declaration directly from the president, without going through the governor of the state. FEMA accepted comments on a draft Tribal Declaration Pilot Guidance through August 2014.[24]

▶ Disaster Relief and Disaster Declarations

Tracing the history of disaster declarations in the United States takes us back to 1803. Katz[9(p48)] cites the Congressional Act of 1803 as the first national disaster declaration. This act, the Federal Domestic Disaster Aid Bill, provided relief for merchants in Portsmouth, New Hampshire, following a major fire by suspending the collection of bonds owed to the U.S. government. The approach for the next century or so was similar, that is, individual declarations approved by Congress for federal assistance after specific disasters. By the 1930s, both the Reconstruction Finance Corporation and the Bureau of Public Roads, among other federal agencies, also supported relief for specific disasters.[4,6]

The first, comprehensive legislation to address disaster relief came in 1950 with the passage of the Disaster Relief Act. Signed into law by President Harry Truman, the program required a presidential disaster declaration[5(p8)] and was intended only to "supplement the efforts and available resources of States and local governments."[8] President Truman's 1953 Executive Order 10427 underscored that, "Federal disaster relief provided under this act shall be deemed to be supplementary to relief afforded by State, local, or private agencies and not in substitution therefore; Federal financial contributions for disaster relief shall be conditioned upon reasonable State and local expenditures for such relief; . . ."[9,25] This Executive Order also changed the authorized federal agent from the Housing and Home Finance Administrator to the Federal Civil Defense Administrator.[9,25] While this change grew out of the federal government's response to the Cold War,[5] it is interesting to note that figuring out where in the federal bureaucracy responsibility for disaster relief should reside would be an ongoing issue.

Other shifts in focus and authorizing agency followed this initial legislation. The Disaster Relief Act was amended in 1966 to include authority for federal assistance during recovery, not just during response, as in the 1950 legislation.[8] In 1974, the Disaster Relief Act (PL 93-288) signed by President Nixon amended the original legislation in several key ways. Title II created a program for disaster preparedness that included technical assistance from the federal government as well as grants to support states in their efforts "for the development of plans, programs, and capabilities for disaster preparedness and prevention."[26] Title III, Disaster Assistance Administration, described the process for a presidential disaster declaration (Section 301, p. 146) and called for the appointment of a federal coordinating officer in the area designated for major disaster relief through this process (Section 303,

p. 147). Emergency support teams could be formed to work with this coordinating officer (Section 304, p. 148). This law also addressed federal assistance programs (pp. 153–159) and economic recovery in the affected area (pp. 160–163).

Robert T. Stafford Disaster Relief and Emergency Assistance Act of 1988

The next significant legislation related to disaster declarations was the Robert T. Stafford Disaster Relief and Emergency Assistance Act of 1988 (PL 100-707) that amended the 1974 Disaster Relief Act. This act, now the current source of regulations for disaster declarations, requires that a governor indicate through a formal request that the state is responding to the disaster and that the state lacks sufficient resources for its response.[10] The president may issue two types of declarations: "Emergency" or "Major Disaster." These declarations are defined in **BOX 2-4**.

Disaster relief provided under any presidential declaration is administered by FEMA. Recall that FEMA was created in 1979 by President Carter's Executive Order 12127 in a move to coordinate the federal government's response to public health emergencies.[9]

A presidential disaster declaration means that a state is eligible for specific types of financial, technical, and logistics assistance in the specified local jurisdictions.[27] Individuals may receive assistance directly, local jurisdictions dealing with a major disaster may request grants for hazard mitigation, and local jurisdictions and certain other organizations (e.g., the American Red Cross) may qualify for public assistance for help with removal of debris, repairs to infrastructure, and provision of emergency medical care, food, water, and housing.[27] The Stafford Act also

---

BOX 2-4 Robert T. Stafford Disaster Relief and Emergency Assistance Act: Definitions

Section 103. AMENDMENTS TO TITLE I—Disaster Relief and Emergency Assistance Amendments

(b) DEFINITION OF EMERGENCY.—Section 102(1) is amended to read as follows: "(1) EMERGENCY.—'Emergency' means any occasion or instance for which, in the determination of the President, Federal assistance is needed to supplement State and local efforts and capabilities to save lives and to protect property and public health and safety, or to lessen or avert the threat of a catastrophe in any part of the United States."

(c) DEFINITION OF MAJOR DISASTER.—Section 102(2) is amended to read as follows: "(2) MAJOR DISASTER.—'Major disaster' means any natural catastrophe (including any hurricane, tornado, storm, high water, winddriven water, tidal wave, tsunami, earthquake, volcanic eruption, landslide, mudslide, snowstorm, or drought), or, regardless of cause, any fire, flood, or explosion, in any part of the United States, which in the determination of the President causes damage of sufficient severity and magnitude to warrant major disaster assistance under this Act to supplement the efforts and available resources of States, local governments, and, disaster relief organizations in alleviating the damage, loss, hardship, or suffering caused thereby."

Data from Stafford Act, Public Law 100-707, 11/23/88; 102 STAT. 4689-90; 42 USC 5122 www.gpo.gov/fdsys/pkg/STATUTE-102/pdf/STATUTE-102-Pg4689.pdf

covers reimbursement by the state where the disaster occurred for services provided through mutual aid agreements, as stated in the 1996 Emergency Management Assistance Compact (EMAC; see in the next section). The Stafford Act provides the framework through which FEMA administers disaster relief programs following any disaster declaration.

▶ Legal Considerations in Emergency Preparedness Planning

As this overview of selected key public health emergency preparedness legislation, regulations, and policies illustrates, roles and responsibilities of local, state, and national governments have evolved over time as the nature of public health threats has changed since the early 2000s. Local jurisdictions and the states are responsible for the health and safety of their residents through their police powers, and states do have some authority for emergency preparedness. Yet, the authority for prevention, response, mitigation, and recovery is shaped by federal mandates that guide local and state planning, establish standards, influence relationships, and direct funding.[28] The events of 9/11, coupled with the global threats of severe acute respiratory syndrome (SARS), H1N1, and Ebola, have underscored the federal government's emphasis on national security as an important dimension of public health emergency preparedness. The response to public health emergencies is always local initially, but what local plans look like and how jurisdictions relate to each other during a public health emergency is in part driven by federal laws and regulations.

There are legal tools that enable local and state governments to prepare for and anticipate certain responses during an emergency through planning. Local jurisdictions and states use Mutual Aid Agreements and Memoranda of Understanding in planning to define what they and/or specific agencies will do following a presidential declaration of a major disaster or emergency through the Stafford Act. The purpose of these documents is to identify resources that may be needed from neighboring jurisdictions when local resources have been exhausted and to provide a framework for addressing the important issues such as logistics, liability, and costs for supplies, equipment, and personnel. Whether a jurisdiction provides assistance to another jurisdiction during recovery from a public health emergency is voluntary if there is no presidential declaration.[28(p50)]

Emergency Management Assistance Compact

The EMAC (Public Law No. 104-321) is a nongovernmental interstate mutual aid agreement. Signed into law in 1996, EMAC is administered by the National Emergency Management Association (NEMA), and the 50 states, the District of Columbia, and three territories—the U.S. Virgin Islands, Puerto Rico, and Guam—are part of the Compact.[29] The Compact enables states to share resources, equipment, and personnel, including National Guard members, with a neighboring state once the president has declared a major disaster or emergency. The state requesting assistance is obligated to reimburse the state that provided assistance.[10] The EMAC traces its roots to initiatives within the Southern Governors, Association to support each other during hurricanes, with Hurricane Andrew in 1992 the major impetus for formalizing these relationships.[29] The largest mobilization of resources occurred in 2005 for Hurricanes Katrina in August and Rita in September. EMAC deployed about 66,000 emergency personnel and 46,500 National Guard members over 90,000 square miles, providing helicopter and air support, communications, and advance team, security, and search and rescue personnel, among other resources.[30]

Emergency Use Authorization

The EUA is codified in Section 564 of the Federal Food, Drug, and Cosmetic Act. Under this regulation, the Secretary of Health and Human Services (HHS) may authorize the FDA to allow the use of a particular drug or device in an emergency situation for which it is not approved.[10] The Secretaries of HHS, Homeland Security, and Defense need to establish that there is a significant risk from a chemical, biological, radiological, or nuclear (CBRN) event (see discussion of this topic later in Chapter 12) before the Secretary of HHS declares that an EUA is necessary.[10] Given the potential threat to national security in such an event, both the 2006 Pandemic and All-Hazards Preparedness Act and the 2013 PAHPRA reaffirmed the importance of the development of countermeasures, including drugs and vaccines for pandemics, and fostered conditions to promote the research, development, and manufacturing of such products.

Quarantine and Isolation

Local jurisdictions, states, and the federal government have the authority to issue quarantine and isolation orders to protect the health and safety of residents. These orders restrict the movement of people who have been exposed to a communicable disease (quarantine) or who have symptoms and are presumed to have the communicable disease (isolation). At the local and state levels, this authority is codified in state statutes. At the federal level, this authority is codified in Sections 311, 361, and 362 of the Public Health Service Act. Federal regulations address interstate and foreign quarantine.[10] The list of diseases for which people can be confined dating from 1983 includes cholera, diphtheria, tuberculosis, plague, smallpox, yellow fever, and viral hemorrhagic fevers.[31] Since 2003, three executive orders have modified the list of communicable diseases for which quarantine and isolation may be used. Executive Order 13295 in 2003 added SARS, and Executive Order 13375 in 2005 added influenza viruses that have the potential to cause a pandemic. Finally, Executive Order 13674 in 2014 clarified the reference to SARS.

Protecting the public from communicable diseases is an essential public health service, yet implementation of an isolation or quarantine order is sometimes controversial and raises ethical concerns. At the state level, the 2014 Ebola quarantine case discussed earlier in this chapter highlighted the tension between protecting the public's health and respecting individual rights. Without any symptoms of Ebola, it was hard for the nurse returning from West Africa to accept the Maine quarantine order (see **BOX 2-1**).

As noted earlier, an example of the federal government using its power in this arena came in 2007 when the CDC placed a citizen with a severe form of drug-resistant tuberculosis who had traveled out of the country in isolation upon his return.[32] The individual disregarded both a restriction not to leave the country and an order not to travel back to the country from Europe given his disease. While he later acknowledged that his travel may not have been the best decision, he raised questions about how he was to have been treated in Italy.[9(p149),33]

▶ Legal Preparedness

Legal preparedness is the idea that practitioners and organizations have the knowledge about legal authorities for public health practice in their jurisdictions and the capability to act in appropriate ways based on existing laws and regulations. The expectation is that laws would be clear, lines of communication open, and actions needed in response to a particular public health event apparent. The reality is that legal issues involving the public's health are complex, and laws and statutes vary greatly among the states. During public health emergencies, this lack of coordination and standards is particularly problematic when lives and damage to property and the environment are at stake. As part of a broader initiative to strengthen public health systems, the Robert Wood Johnson Foundation and the W.K. Kellogg Foundation funded the Turning Point program, which included a national collaborative on modernization of public health statutes.[34] The model statute that local, state, and tribal governments could use to enhance their legal preparedness was issued in 2003, and as of August 2007, 48 out of 133 bills in 33 states had passed.[35] This work reflects a concerted effort to address what was acknowledged to be a gap in the public health infrastructure.

Particularly since 9/11, public health emergency legal preparedness has taken on more urgency. Our experience since 2001 with diseases such as SARS, H1N1, and, most recently, Ebola underscores the importance of clear lines of authority and mechanisms for assistance across jurisdictions. The Model State Emergency Health Powers Act was issued in 2001, and as of July 2006, 38 states had passed 66 bills that adopted language from the Act.[35] This work prompted considerable discussion about the role of the federal and state governments during public health emergencies as well as the need to balance the rights of individuals during periods of crisis when the health and safety of the public are of paramount importance.[9]

Along with work to modernize statutes related to public health emergency legal preparedness, efforts have been under way more generally to define gaps in legal preparedness for emergencies and to identify the key components of legal preparedness and the competencies necessary for the public health workforce. Four core elements were identified in a 2007 summit designed to address legal preparedness: laws and legal authorities, competency in using laws effectively, coordination of legal interventions across jurisdictions and sectors, and information on laws and best practices.[36] These core elements provide a framework for public health practitioners and local and state leaders to examine local practices and conditions, identify gaps, and create solutions to enhance legal preparedness during public health emergencies. To assist jurisdictions in this work, the National Association of County and City Health Officials (NACCHO) has developed an emergency preparedness training kit.[37]

With respect to competencies for educating and training the public health workforce to know how to use the laws effectively, the CDC and the Association of Schools and Programs of Public Health (ASPPH) developed the Public Health Emergency Law Competency Model in 2008 for mid-tier professionals.[38] The competencies address three domains: (1) systems preparedness and response, (2) management and protection of property and supplies, and (3) management and protection of persons. Of particular importance is the focus on a systems approach to emergency legal preparedness, as reflected in Domain 1. Having the knowledge and information about laws related to emergencies, coordinating and communicating with partners, and acting within the scope of the specific legal authorities are essential in all phases of public health emergency preparedness planning, prevention, response, and recovery.

▶ Conclusion

In the U.S. history of public health emergency response to both man-made and natural disasters, legislation, regulations, and presidential directives reflect the federal government's evolving policies toward prevention, mitigation, response, and recovery. While the response to disasters has always been driven at the local level, the federal government's role in the face of external events has become more centralized with respect to the articulation of a national preparedness goal and a national response plan for all phases of an emergency event. Initially, federal assistance was only provided during the recovery phase, as local jurisdictions managed to the best of their capabilities during the event. Various revisions to disaster declaration legislation now provide governors the opportunity through the Robert T. Stafford Act to request aid during the response to a disaster. Organizational structures changed over time as leaders struggled with how best to manage the response and support recovery with logistics and financial assistance. From the establishment of FEMA in 1979 via Executive Order 12127 to the creation of the DHS in the Homeland Security Act of 2002 and FEMA's more prominent role in disaster management, the federal government sought a more unified vision for ensuring domestic security and safety. Emergency preparedness planning was mandated at all levels, sometimes with specific approaches in mind. Pets and service animals, for example, were the priority in the PETS Act of 2006 following the experiences of Hurricane Katrina in 2005. The PAHPRA of 2013 mandated that protection of children and vulnerable populations be addressed in grantees' All-Hazards Public Health Emergency Preparedness and Response plans.

No one law, executive order, regulation, or directive can anticipate all the possible outcomes from either a man-made or natural disaster. Timing, scope, and complexity of the event affect the nature of response and recovery at all levels. The events of 9/11, the anthrax letters, and Hurricanes Katrina, Rita, and Sandy marked significant turning points in how the United States addresses emergency preparedness. There will always be a need to evaluate how laws work and what plans need further coordination and practice. While the federal government seeks an integrated approach to response and recovery using a whole-of-government and the whole community framework, public health law is an integral part of the infrastructure. Though the mission of public health embodies a social justice lens, the realities of the social, political, and economic environment at the local, state, and federal levels mean that legal preparedness needs to be a part of our ongoing approach to ensure a fair and equitable, coordinated, and comprehensive approach to prevention, response, mitigation, and recovery from a man-made or natural disaster.

Discussion Questions

1. Review the information about the quarantine case involving the nurse who returned to the United States from treating West African patients with Ebola in October 2014. Do you agree with her decision to challenge both the New Jersey and Maine quarantine orders? Why or why not? Do you agree with Judge Charles LaVerdiere's decision in the Maine case? Why or why not?
2. Do you believe there should be more or less federal involvement in state and local disaster response? Explain your response.

3. Which laws answer the question, "Who is in charge?" How might we evaluate the impact of these laws?
4. What documents and/or legislation describe the roles of nongovernmental agencies in an emergency? How are these relationships defined?
5. What issues was the Post-Katrina Emergency Management Reform Act of 2006 intended to address? What evidence, if any, is there that the legislative solutions to challenges faced during Hurricane Katrina have been effective?

References

1. Turnock BJ. *Public Health: What It Is and How It Works*. 5th ed. Burlington, MA: Jones & Bartlett Learning; 2012.
2. Dexter B. Mayhew V. Hickox: Balancing Maine's public's health with personal liberties during the Ebola "Crisis". *Maine Law Review*. Available at www.mainelawreview.org/volume-68-no-1-2016/mayhew-v-hickox/. Accessed November 2, 2014.
3. Cornish A. Is it legal to Quarantine someone who's not sick? *National Public Radio*. October 30, 2014. Available at http://www.npr.org/2014/10/30/360179363/is-it-legal-to-quarantine-someone-whos-not-sick. Accessed November 2, 2014.
4. Federal Emergency Management Agency (FEMA). History. Allgov.com. Available at www.allgov.com/departments/department-of-homeland-security/federal-emergency-management-agency-fema?agencyid=7345. Accessed October 31, 2014.
5. Mener AS. Disaster response in the United States of America: an analysis of the bureaucratic and political history of a failing system. *CUREJ: College Undergraduate Research Electronic Journal*. University of Pennsylvania. May 10, 2007. Available at http://repository.upenn.edu/curej/63.
6. FEMA. About the agency. Available at https://www.fema.gov/about-agency. Updated August 2014. Accessed October 19, 2014.
7. Executive Order 12127—Federal Emergency Management Agency. 1-102. 3 C.F.R. 376. March 31, 1979. Available at https://fas.org/irp/offdocs/eo/eo-12127.htm. Accessed November 9, 2014.
8. Baca AM. History of disaster legislation. FEMA. *On Call*. September 1, 2008. Accessed October 19, 2014.
9. Katz R. *Essentials of Public Health Preparedness*. Burlington, MA: Jones & Bartlett Learning; 2013.
10. Kershner S. Selected federal legal authorities pertinent to public health emergencies. Centers for Disease Control and Prevention, Public Health Law Program. Available at https://www.cdc.gov/phlp/docs/ph-emergencies.pdf. Updated 2014. Accessed November 9, 2014.
11. Public Health Security and Bioterrorism Preparedness and Response Act. 116 STAT. 594, 42 USC 201. Available at http://www.gpo.gov/fdsys/pkg/PLAW-107publ188/pdf/PLAW-107publ188.pdf. Accessed December 7, 2014.
12. Public Health Security and Bioterrorism Preparedness and Response Act. 116 STAT. 596, 42 USC 201. Available at http://www.gpo.gov/fdsys/pkg/PLAW-107publ188/pdf/PLAW-107publ188.pdf. Accessed December 7, 2014.
13. Homeland security presidential directive 5: management of domestic incidents. *The White House*. February 28, 2003. Available at http://www.dhs.gov/sites/default/files/publications/Homeland Security Presidential Directive 5.pdf. Accessed December 14, 2014.
14. Homeland security presidential directive-8: national preparedness. *The White House*. December 17, 2003. Available at fas.org/irp/offdocs/nspd/nspd-8.html. Accessed December 14, 2014.
15. American State & Territorial Health Officials. Emergency Use Authorization Toolkit, Public Readiness & Emergency Preparedness Act Fact Sheet: How The Law Works. Compiled 2011. Available at http://www.astho.org/Programs/Preparedness/Public-Health-Emergency-Law/Emergency-Use-Authorization-Toolkit/Public-Readiness-and-Emergency-Preparedness-Act-Fact-Sheet/. Accessed January 4, 2015.

16. U.S. Department of Health and Human Services. Office of the assistant secretary for preparedness & response. Public Readiness & Emergency Preparedness Act. Available at http://www.phe.gov/preparedness/legal/prepact/pages/default.aspx. Reviewed December 9, 2014. Accessed January 4, 2015.

17. U.S. Department of Health and Human Services. Office of the assistant secretary for preparedness & response. Public Readiness & Emergency Preparedness Act. Current declarations. Available at https://www.phe.gov/Preparedness/legal/prepact/Pages/default .aspx. Last Reviewed May 10, 2017. Accessed September 1, 2017.

18. Legal Information Institute. Public health and medical preparedness and response functions. 42 U.S. Code 2801 §300hh. Available at https://www.gpo.gov/fdsys/pkg/STATUTE-120/html /STATUTE-120-Pg2831.htm. Accessed September 1, 2017.

19. Public Law 109-417. December 6, 2006. 120 STAT. 2846. Available at https://www.gpo.gov /fdsys/pkg/PLAW-109publ417/pdf/PLAW-109publ417.pdf. Accessed September 1, 2017.

20. Public Law 109-308. October 6, 2006. 120 STAT. 1725-26. Available at http://www.gpo.gov /fdsys/pkg/PLAW-109publ308/pdf/PLAW-109publ308.pdf. Accessed January 4, 2015.

21. Simon S. A bipartisan bill helped save pets from Harvey, and maybe their humans too. National Public Radio. *Weekend Edition Saturday*. Published September 2, 2017. Available at http://www.npr.org/2017/09/02/547972616/a-bipartisan-bill-helped-save-pets-from-harvey-and -maybe-their-humans-too. Accessed September 2, 2017.

22. Lurie N. US Department of Health and Human Services. Statement on the Pandemic & All Hazards Preparedness Reauthorization Act. March 13, 2013. Revised August 2013. Available at http://www.hhs.gov/news/press/2013pres/03/20130313a.html. Accessed January 8, 2015.

23. FEMA. Sandy Recovery Improvement Act of 2013. Available at https://www.fema.gov /sandy-recovery-improvement-act-2013. Updated December 3, 2014. Accessed January 4, 2015.

24. FEMA. Consultation on disaster declaration process for tribes. Available at http://www .fema.gov/consultation-disaster-declaration-process-tribes. Updated August 8, 2014. Accessed January 4, 2015.

25. Executive Order 10427. Administration of disaster relief. The American Presidency Project. Harry S. Truman. January 16, 1953 Available at http://www.presidency.ucsb.edu/ws/?pid=78522. Accessed October 26, 2014.

26. Public Law 93-288. Disaster Relief Act Amendments of 1974. May 21, 1974. 88 STAT. 145. Available at http://uscode.house.gov/statutes/pl/93/288.pdf. Accessed October 26, 2014.

27. Association of State and Territorial Health Officers. Emergency authority and immunity toolkit. 2014. Available at http://www.astho.org/Programs/Preparedness/Public-Health -Emergency-Law/Emergency-Authority-and-Immunity-Toolkit/Emergency-Authority-and -Immunity-Toolkit/. Accessed November 2, 2014.

28. Landesman LY. *Public Health Management of Disasters: The Practice Guide*. 3rd ed. Washington, DC: APHA Press; 2012.

29. Emergency Management Assistance Compact. 1996. Available at https://www.emacweb .org/index.php/learn-about-emac/emac-history. Accessed January 18, 2015.

30. Copple A. EMAC Overview. August 2006. Slide 31. Available at https://www.fema.gov /media-library-data/20130726-1726-25045-0915/060802emac.pdf. Accessed September 2, 2017.

31. Centers for Disease Control and Prevention. Quarantine and isolation. Available at https://www.cdc.gov/quarantine/index.html. Updated May 30, 2014. Accessed January 18, 2015.

32. Altman LK. TB Patient isolated after taking two flights. *New York Times*. Published May 30, 2007. Available at http://query.nytimes.com/gst/fullpage.html?res=9403E5DA1430F933A05756 C0A9619C8B63. Accessed November 23, 2014.

33. Schwartz J. Tangle of conflicting accounts in TB Patient's Odyssey. *New York Times*. Published June 2, 2007. Available at http://www.nytimes.com/2007/06/02/health/02tick.html. Accessed January 15, 2015.

34. Robert Wood Johnson Foundation. Turning point: collaborating for a new century in public health. Published May 13, 2008. Available at http://www.rwjf.org/content/dam/farm /reports/program_results_reports/2008/rwjf69892. Accessed January 18, 2015.

35. Centers for Law and the Public's Health. Collaborative at Johns Hopkins and Georgetown Universities. The Turning Point Model State Public Health Act (MSPHA). Published 2008.

Available at http://www.publichealthlaw.net/ModelLaws/MSPHA.php. Updated January 27, 2010. Accessed January 18, 2015.

36. Benjamin GC, Moulton AD. Public health legal preparedness: a framework for action. *Journal of Law, Medicine & Ethics*. 2008;36:13–17. doi:10.1111/j.1748-720X.2008.00254.x.

37. National Association of County and City Health Officials. Public health and the law: an emergency preparedness training kit. Published 2012.

38. Centers for Disease Control and Prevention. Public Health Law Program. *The Public Health Emergency Law Competency Model*. Updated March 17, 2014. Available at https://www.cdc.gov/phlp/publications/topic/phel-competencies.html. Accessed January 18, 2015.

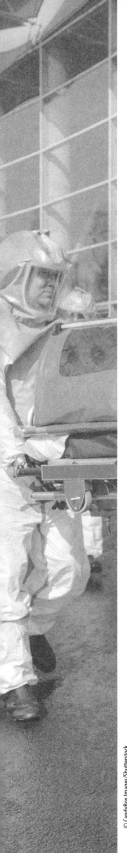

PART II
Hazards and Threats

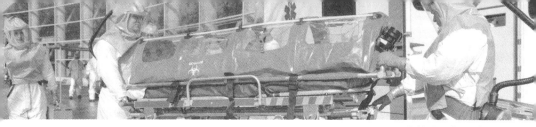

CHAPTER 3

Chemical, Biological, Radiological, Nuclear, and Explosive (CBRNE) Events

LEARNING OBJECTIVES

By the end of this chapter, readers should be able to:

- Define chemical, biological, radiological, nuclear, and explosive (CBRNE) events
- Understand the varying impacts that CBRNE incidents have on populations and their health
- Understand the multiple causes of CBRNE incidents
- Distinguish the difference between chemical and biological agents and radiological and nuclear devices

▶ Introduction

Within the past two or so decades, events such as the Aum Shinrikyo Tokyo subway sarin gas attack in March 1995, the New York and Washington, DC, anthrax attacks in October 2001, the Madrid train bombings in March 2004, the Fukushima Daiichi nuclear meltdown in March 2011 following the Tōhoku earthquake and tsunami, the Boston Marathon bombing in April 2013, the West Texas fertilizer plant explosion in 2013, and the West Virginia CSX train derailment and explosion in February 2015 are stark, vivid reminders of the reality of biological, chemical, radiological, nuclear, or explosive disasters or attacks.

Whether in the United States or abroad, whether triggered naturally by a disaster or perpetrated intentionally by individuals or groups, these events constitute a particular threat that requires coordinated surveillance efforts, careful planning, and coordinated response operations among a range of local, state, and national partners. As the examples reveal, such an event may constitute a terrorist attack or may be the result of a technological disaster.

The role of public health in CBRNE events involves surveillance, planning, partnership, and carefully coordinated response operations. While the public health role in any CBRNE event is significant, public health practitioners must partner with a range of governmental, community, and private entities, all of whom will be needed to ensure a comprehensive and coordinated response to these complex threats.

▶ Chemical Agents

Chemical agents are manufactured compounds that have harmful effects on humans, varying with their route of transmission and which human system is affected. Routes of transmission can be inhalational or through the skin. Human exposure to chemical agents must be mediated quickly with appropriate countermeasures to minimize the harmful effects of these agents. The Centers for Disease Control and Prevention (CDC) identify several categories of chemical agents. Four of these categories stand out as the most threatening because of their use in warfare or terrorist attacks: blister, blood, choking or lung, and nerve agents.[1] Chemical emergencies occur when any of these chemical materials are released in a manner that could cause harm to the health of populations. As we have seen in recent history, chemical emergencies can be the result of intentional acts, terrorism, or accidental events.[2]

Blister Agents

Blister agents, or vesicants, affect the skin, eyes, lungs, and digestive track. The most well-known blister agents are lewisite and mustard gas, both of which cause pain, swelling, and tearing of the eyes, sneezing and runny nose, cough and shortness of breath, diarrhea and vomiting, and redness and blistering of the skin.[3,4] In the case of mustard gas, the blisters are yellow.[3] Both lewisite and mustard gas were originally developed for use during wartime. Lewisite came too late in World War I for it to have been used. Mustard gas, meanwhile, was used in World Wars I and II, while the Italians used it against Ethiopia in 1936. It was also used in the Iran–Iraq war during the 1980s.[5,6] Since the 2011 outbreak of conflict in Syria, it is estimated that at least 984 people have been killed in attacks with chemical and toxic substances.[7] More recently, mustard gas has been used by the Islamic State in northern Syria.[8] Neither lewisite nor mustard gas occurs naturally in the environment, and there are no medical uses for either chemical agent. This fact lends knowledge to law enforcement authorities and emergency planners that an incident utilizing either of these two agents, aside from an unintentional spill, could likely be the result of terrorist activity.

Blood Agents

Blood agents affect the blood. The most well-known blood agent is cyanide, of which there are four types. Hydrogen cyanide (HC) and cyanogen chloride are colorless gases, while sodium cyanide or potassium cyanide are crystals.[9] Breathing cyanide, absorbing it through the skin, or eating foods with it causes dizziness, headache, nausea/vomiting, rapid breathing, rapid heart rate, and/or restlessness, as cells cannot use oxygen. In serious cases of exposure, loss of consciousness can occur. The heart and brain are most affected by cyanide since these organs depend on oxygen.[9] Cyanide has also been used in wartime. Germany used HC as Zyklon B in the extermination camps during World War II, and cyanide is among the chemical agents thought to have been used by Iraq in Halabja against the Kurds in 1988.[6,10] Cyanide occurs both naturally and industrially. Plants such as lima beans and almonds produce cyanide, and the pits of apricots and peaches can release chemicals that make cyanide. In industry, cyanide is used in the manufacturing of plastics, paper, and textiles and is found in cigarette smoke.[9]

FIGURE 3-1 depicts the National Fire Protection Association (NFPA) symbol for HC. HC is a colorless or pale blue substance. Its slight odor does not give an indication of a dangerous chemical. As a result, persons exposed to HC may not readily know of exposure to the chemical. Because HC is a highly systemic asphyxiant chemical, meaning it can affect the major systems throughout the entire body very quickly, exposure to HC must be treated quickly. The NFPA symbol provides appropriate warnings of the symptoms of HC exposure. The color coding of the symbol also provides an indication of the various dangers associated with HC exposure, including health dangers, flammability, reactivity, and other special considerations. The color codes also provide indications to first responders of the types of personal protective equipment that should be utilized when working in areas contaminated with HC.[9]

Choking Agents

Choking agents affect the nose, throat, and lungs through damage to the respiratory system. Examples of choking or lung agents include ammonia, chlorine, and

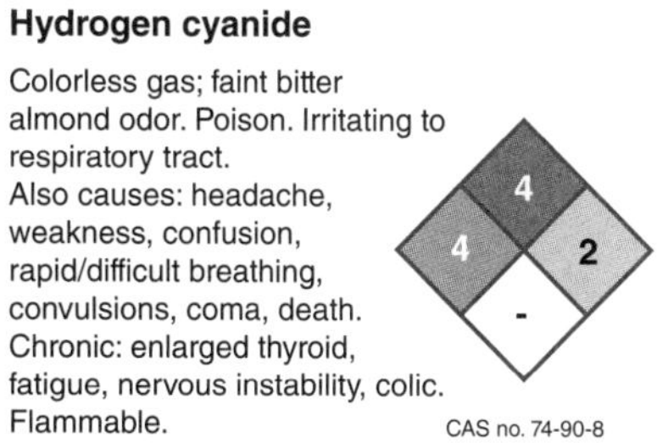

Hydrogen cyanide

Colorless gas; faint bitter almond odor. Poison. Irritating to respiratory tract.
Also causes: headache, weakness, confusion, rapid/difficult breathing, convulsions, coma, death.
Chronic: enlarged thyroid, fatigue, nervous instability, colic. Flammable.

CAS no. 74-90-8

FIGURE 3-1 National Fire Protection Association 704 Signal/Hydrogen Cyanide. Health/Blue = 4; Flammability/Red = 4; Reactivity/Yellow = 2; Special/White

Data from Chemicals G – N. MySafetyLabels.com. Google Images. Accessed July 17, 2015. CDC, National Institute for Occupational Safety and Health. Hydrogen Cyanide (AC): Systemic Agent. Available at: www.cdc.gov/niosh/ershdb/emergencyresponsecard_29750038.html. Updated June 1, 2015. Accessed July 17, 2015.

phosgene. Chlorine has a yellow-green color and strong odor of bleach, while phosgene ranges from colorless to pale yellow with a strong odor in high amounts.[11] Among the symptoms caused by these gases are watery eyes and blurred vision, difficulty breathing, nausea and vomiting, and fluid in the lungs.

Choking agents were the first chemical weapons used in battle. As chlorine and phosgene settle in low areas, these gases were effective in the trenches of World War I; a large majority of the deaths were caused by phosgene.[12] Between 1915 and 1918, first the Germans, then the British, and finally, the United States used chlorine and phosgene.[6,12] The "successful" use of these agents resulted in the development of expanded chemical weapons programs.[6,13]

The most deadly chemical accident worldwide involved the choking agent methyl isocyanate. On December 3, 1984, in Bhopal, India, a Union Carbide pesticide factory leaked about 40 tons of this chemical, killing between 3000 and 5000 immediately, injuring thousands, and affecting thousands more with various health effects in the 30-plus years since then.[14] While Union Carbide paid a settlement of $470 million in 1989 to the Indian government, there has been only limited cleanup of the site of the abandoned plant, and there is no scientific evidence about the health effects of contaminated water in the area.[15] Dow Chemical acquired Union Carbide in 2001, and responsibility for who should pay for the cleanup remains mired in the Indian courts. Meanwhile, local nongovernmental agencies provide resources to help families address very challenging situations.

Several choking agents are used in industry. Methyl isocyanate and phosgene are used in the manufacture of pesticides. Chlorine has a wide range of manufacturing applications (bleach in production of paper and cloth, household cleaning products; pesticides, rubber, solvents) and treatment applications (swimming pools, water treatments; industrial waste and sewage treatment).[11,12]

Nerve Agents

Nerve agents affect the nervous system by overstimulating the production of the enzyme acetylcholine and thereby speeding up the respiratory system and muscle contractions. Examples of nerve agents are sarin, tabun, soman, and VX, all tasteless liquids that become vaporized through heating or evaporation. These chemical agents cause symptoms ranging from tearing eyes, runny nose, blurred vision, chest tightness, diarrhea, confusion, and slow or fast heart rate to convulsions, paralysis, and possibly death.[16] Although nerve agents are classified as organophosphates, like the pesticides/herbicides parathion, malathion, and diazinon, they are highly toxic, man-made chemical warfare agents. Sarin, tabun, and soman were originally developed as pesticides by Germany in the 1930s and 1940s, while VX was developed by England in the 1950s.[16,17] There is evidence that nerve agents were used during the Iran–Iraq war in the 1980s, with the most documented instance thought to be the March 16, 1988, Iraqi attack on Halabja, a Kurdish city near the Iranian border.[10,17] In addition to mustard gas, Saddam Hussein's forces likely dropped sarin and tabun on the city.

Aum Shinrikyo's intentional release of sarin in the Tokyo subway on March 20, 1995, is the most compelling example of a terrorist attack using a nerve agent.

Aum Shinrikyo, which means "Supreme Truth," had about 40,000 members at this time, and it is known that Japanese authorities were planning a raid on the headquarters in light of other suspicious activities.[18] Members of this group placed five wrapped packages in the stations of three subway lines and punctured them with umbrella tips, allowing the liquid to seep out.[18] Twelve people died, and thousands were injured. Many more people would have died had Aum Shinrikyo's leaders been able to figure out a better way to release the gas. The challenge in preventing such attacks is coordinating surveillance of suspicious activities by fringe groups across a range of partners. Advances in technology and access to the Internet put toxic agents in the hands of people who are no longer dependent on specialized training for skills in creating and using lethal weapons.[18]

The role of public health officials in response to a chemical terrorism attack includes communication to hospitals and healthcare partners when a chemical attack has been identified. This communication should include the location, scope, and severity of the attack, as well as known or suspected impacts on the healthcare delivery system. Public health officials will also need to provide any special treatment recommendations to hospitals and necessary laboratory testing, and ensure fast, efficient, situational awareness to healthcare and other public safety partners. Proper situational awareness ensures that rapidly changing conditions are effectively communicated, so that response actions can be modified quickly. Public health's role also includes planning that identifies the most effective and efficient manner to deliver medical countermeasures (chemical antidotes) to those affected by the attack. Treatment of chemical exposures is extremely time sensitive; chemical antidotes must be administered within hours of the exposure in order to be effective. This means public health must closely coordinate with hospitals to ensure the availability of countermeasures for treatment purposes. Due to the time constraints associated with the treatment of chemical exposures, antidotes should be readily available at hospitals or quickly delivered to hospitals to maximize effectiveness of the treatment. Several jurisdictions across the United States have achieved this capability through partnership with the CDC and participation in the CHEMPACK program.

The CHEMPACK Program

The CHEMPACK program was established in 2003 to provide the forward placement of critical nerve agent medicines around the country. According to the CDC, the CHEMPACK program resources can reach about 90% of the U.S. population within 1 hour, or nearly everyone in the country within a few minutes to less than 2 hours of recognition of the need for these medicines.[19] One thousand three hundred and forty (1340) locations around the country monitor and maintain 1960 containers with medicines and supplies.[19] Most of the locations, or cache sites, are hospitals and fire stations, and first responders work with local and state public health partners in coordinating planning as well as training and exercises.

While CDC administers the CHEMPACK program, local and state health departments manage the local/state planning process and coordinate program oversight and implementation. **TABLE 3-1** summarizes the responsibilities of CDC and the states or localities.

TABLE 3-1 The CHEMPACK Program: CDC and Local/State Health Department Responsibilities

CDC	Local/State Health Department
Ownership of nerve agent antidotes/assets	Coordination of distribution of nerve agent antidotes/assets within state or locality
Approval of site locations	Oversight of receipt, storage, maintenance, monitoring, reporting and activation
Implementation of periodic site visits	Coordination of site visits
Administration of Shelf Life Extension Program (SLEP) with Department of Defense and Food and Drug Administration	Review/updating of state/local CHEMPACK plan
	Provision and coordination of annual training, exercising, and evaluating requirements

Effective planning and preparedness for response with chemical medical countermeasures includes close coordination between CDC, state, regional, and local partners. Among the partners are regional hospital preparedness coalitions, hospitals, regional and local emergency medical services (EMS), local police, and local and state public health officials. Strong relationships at all levels are important for ensuring good communications flow for planning and response, as the decision to send the antidotes to the field or a particular hospital is made locally.

The CHEMPACK program addresses not only the issue of a location's distance and time from medical resources during an emergency event, but also the issue of availability of an ample supply of appropriate nerve agent antidotes (**FIGURE 3-2**). Hospitals and pharmacies do not stock the amount of antidotes that would be needed to treat victims of a nerve agent attack or large-scale unintentional release. Three antidotes are used to treat the symptoms caused by nerve agents: atropine sulfate, Pralidoxime, and diazepam. Atropine sulfate slows the tearing of the eyes and nose as well as diarrhea and vomiting, while Pralidoxime or "2-PAM" lowers blood pressure, slows the heart rate, and reduces muscle weakness and paralysis. The third drug, diazepam, reduces convulsions.[20]

The wire-mesh CHEMPACK containers are specially configured with nerve agent antidotes for quick deployment in the field and in the hospital setting. Each CHEMPACK location has both EMS and hospital containers. The EMS containers include auto-injectors that are easier to use at the scene of an emergency incident. Up to 454 people can be treated with these supplies. The hospital containers have multi-use vials for dosing and long-term care, and up to 1000 patients can be treated with these supplies. The nerve agent antidotes are packaged in smaller boxes with

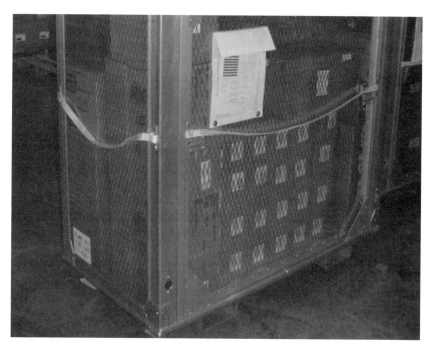

FIGURE 3-2 CHEMPACK container

Reproduced from U.S. Centers for Disease Control. *Public Health Matters* Blog. February 19, 2015. CDC's CHEMPACK Program — The Stockpile that may protect you from a chemical attack. Available at: www.blogs.cdc.gov/publichealthmatters/2015/02 /cdcs-chempack-program-the-stockpile-that-may-protect-you-from-a-chemical-attack/ Accessed: November 15, 2015.

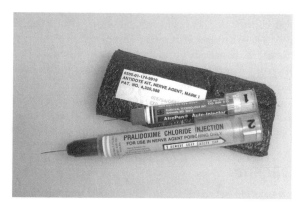

FIGURE 3-3 Atropine and pralidoxime chloride (2-PAM) auto-injectors from CHEMPACK EMS Container

© Greg Mathieson/REX/Shutterstock.

color-coded tags for easy transfer to the field, other hospitals, or to the emergency room on-site at the host hospital. Local plans and protocols define partner roles and responsibilities and procedures for activation and transport of the CHEMPACK assets during an emergency event (**FIGURE 3-3**).

Due to the value of these critical medical countermeasures, local, state, and federal officials all play a role in securing the safety and integrity of these drugs.

Local and state officials are responsible for identifying all deployment or storing locations (i.e., hospitals and EMS provider locations). These officials are also responsible for development of appropriate plans for further breakdown and transport of these assets from storing locations to nonstoring locations; these assets are very expensive and are not sufficient in quantity to afford deployment to all hospitals and EMS locations across the country; therefore, local and state officials must strategically place assets in locations that are easily accessible, yet also have the capability to conduct further breakdown for shipment to other locations. Federal government officials (CDC) take responsibility for electronic monitoring of these medications on a 24/7/365 basis. All CHEMPACK containers are electronically wired, in their storing locations, which provides CDC with the capacity to monitor temperature and security of the assets. Chemical antidotes are temperature sensitive; thus, it is important to ensure that proper temperature ranges are maintained at all times. Electronic sensors will trigger security alarms to the CDC anytime the CHEMPACK temperature gauges begin to fluctuate to dangerously high or low temperatures. Sensors will also trigger alarms to the CDC when the physical security of the containers has been compromised. Upon receipt of an alarm, CDC officials will notify local or state public health and emergency management officials, who in turn work locally with officials at storing locations to determine the origin of the temperature or security breach and work to mitigate the problem. Local and state officials, therefore, must ensure that up-to-date contact information for responsible parties at storing locations is maintained at all times.

The threat from chemical agents is real. Examples of intentional and unintentional releases of toxic chemicals reveal the magnitude of harm to people and communities that is possible, with consequences felt for decades after. In the short term, these events can cause fear, chaos, and large surges on the healthcare delivery system. Longer-term effects include lingering health effects on persons exposed to chemical agents.[6] The Chemical Weapons Convention, enacted in 1997, provides a framework for member nations to prohibit the use and production of chemical weapons. The treaty, formally known as the Convention on the Prohibition of the Development, Production, Stockpiling and Use of Chemical Weapons and on their Destruction, obligates members to prohibit the use and production of chemical weapons, as well as the destruction of all current chemical weapons under the control of a member state or nation.[21]

Biological Agents

Biological agents are viruses, bacteria, or other germs that have been weaponized for intentional use against humans, plants, or animals.[7] The intentional release of biological agents is intended to cause injury, illness, or death within populations for the sole purpose of inciting fear and chaos. Biological agents are spread through the air, food, or water and can be transmitted to humans via inhalation or ingestion into the body, or through the skin.[22] These agents are inexpensive to obtain, some occur naturally in the environment, and they are relatively easy to weaponize and disseminate.

Bioterrorism agents are divided into three categories: Category A, B, and C agents. Categorization is based on the lethality and impact of these agents, their ability to cause disease, and ease of spread as weapons.[22]

Category A Agents

Category A agents cause the greatest amount of concern. These agents pose the highest risk to the public's health and are considered to be the highest threats. Category A agents primarily occur in nature but can be weaponized and delivered relatively easily for malicious intent. The major concern with Category A agents includes the fact that they:

- Can be easily transmitted via person-to-person contact
- Can cause high rates of illness and death (public health concern)
- Can cause a large degree of public panic and chaos
- Require specific preparedness actions[22]

Category A agents are those that have the best potential to cause the greatest amount of morbidity and mortality. These agents are also fairly stable in the environment and thus can be readily spread nondescriptly to cause disease or other harm. Additionally, great harm can be caused to large numbers of people utilizing small amounts of these disease agents. **TABLE 3-2** depicts the Category A agents.

TABLE 3-2 Category A Biological Agents[23]

Agent (Disease Caused)	Lethality (Likely to Cause Death)	Incubation Period	Effective Dose	Environmental Stability
Bascillus anthracis (Anthrax)	High	1–6 days	10,000–50,000 spores	Very stable for many years
Yersinia pestis (Plague)	High	1–6 days	100–500 organisms	Stable for 1 year
Variola major (Smallpox)	High	7–17 days	10–100 organisms	Very stable
Clostridium botulinum (Botulism)	High	1–5 days	0.001 mcg/kg weight	Relatively stable
Francisella tularensis (Tularemia)	Low	2–15 days	10–50 organisms	Stable for months
Viral hemorraghic fevers (Ebola, Marburg, Lassa, etc.)	High	2–6 days	10–100 organisms	Unstable

TABLE 3-3 Category B Biological Agents[24]

Agent (Disease Caused)	Lethality (Likely to Cause Death)	Incubation Period	Effective Dose	Environmental Stability
Burkholderia pseudomallei (Meliodosis)		1–21 days		Stable for years
Coxiella burnetti (Q Fever)	Low	15–40 days	1–10 organisms	Stable for months
Brucella species (Brucellosis)	Low	Months	10–100 organisms	Very stable
Burkholderia mallei (Glanders)				Stable for months
Staphylococcus enterotoxin B	Moderate	Less than 1 day	0.03 mcg	Moderately stable
Rickettsia prowazeki (Typhus fever)				

Data from *Bioterrorism and Biological Warfare Agents* www.immed.org/illness/bioterrorism.html and B. Mallei and B. Pseudomallei as Bioterrorism Agents.[29] www.ima.org.il/FilesUpload/IMAJ/0/46/23087.pdf

Category B Agents

Category B agents are the second highest category of biological agents (**TABLE 3-3**). Category B agents are of less concern than Category A agents. Characteristics of Category B agents include the following:

- They are moderately easy to spread.
- They result in moderate illness rates and low death rates.
- They require specific enhancements of CDC's laboratory capacity and enhanced disease monitoring.[22]

Category C Agents

The third category of biological agents is the Category C agents. These third-priority agents consist of viruses and organisms that are emerging diseases that could be engineered for malicious purposes. Category C agents:

- Are easily available
- Are easily produced and spread
- Have a high potential for morbidity and mortality

Category C agents include:[25]

- Nipah virus
- Hantaviruses
- Tickborne hemorrhagic fever viruses
- Tickborne encephalitis viruses
- Yellow fever
- Multidrug-resistant tuberculosis

Radiological and Nuclear Explosive Events

Radiological and nuclear events result from the detonation or explosion of a device containing radiological or nuclear material. These events can be terrorism events or unfortunate accidents. A radiological emergency is characterized by the exposure to the release of radiological material, whereas nuclear emergencies are characterized by blasts or explosions in which nuclear material is widely spread.[26,27]

While some radiological and nuclear events can be accidental, such as unintentional exposure to high levels of radiological material in the healthcare setting, those that are most concerning are those that are terrorist in nature. From the terrorism perspective, radiological and nuclear events are classified into four threat categories:

- Detonation of a dirty bomb or radiological dispersal device using radioactive material
- Attack of a nuclear facility (power plant or waste storage site)
- Theft of a nuclear weapon by a nonstate actor
- Development of an improvised nuclear device using nuclear material[28]

Radiological and nuclear events are low probability events but remain a top concern due to poor relationships between the United States and non-ally nation-states across the world. Short of the launch of a nuclear missile aimed at the United States, it is generally accepted that nuclear terrorism events are unlikely to occur. That is due to the fact that nuclear weapons across the world are not abundant and tend to be heavily guarded and not fully assembled.[29] However, radiological materials are relatively abundant due to commercial uses and, therefore, are more easily obtained.[28] Radiological materials can be constructed into bombs or dispersal devices and used to cause harm. **FIGURE 3-4** illustrates the components of an improvised explosive device.

In the event that a radiological or nuclear event does occur, first responders will be responsible for cleanup of the radioactive material, including robust decontamination efforts. Public health responders will be responsible for providing medical countermeasures to counteract the health effects of the hazardous material.

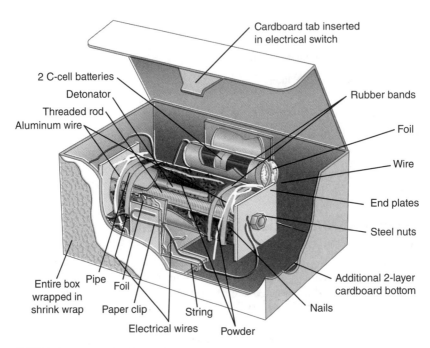

FIGURE 3-4 Improvised explosive device

Data from Global Security.org. Improvised Explosive Devices (IEDs)/Booby Traps. IED Overview. Available at: www.globalsecurity.org /military/intro/ied.htm Accessed: August 31, 2017.

▶ Conclusion

Public health responders face a myriad of threats and vulnerabilities. Acts of terrorism utilizing CBRNE agents are increasingly concerning, largely due to ongoing action on the part of terrorist states and organizations to inflict fear and chaos among the American public. Among the CBRNE events, the threats that pose the greatest risk to national security are the Category A biological agents. These agents are easily acquired, and while they pose danger to those handling them, when actors are successful in altering the genetic characteristics of these organism for the purpose of weaponization, their presence is relatively undetectable until the effects begin to be manifested. It is the responsibility of public health officials and other responders not only to know and understand the consequences of all CBRNE threats, but also to develop plans and processes for protecting the public from these threats.

Discussion Questions

1. What are CBRNE emergencies?
2. Are the effects of chemical agent exposure experienced quickly or after a period of time has occurred?
3. What is the value of the CHEMPACK program? Why is it important for chemical antidotes to be forward deployed to healthcare facilities?

4. What are the three categories of biological agents? Which of the three categories are of greatest concern to preparedness and response officials? Why?
5. Define a radiological event. Now define a nuclear event. Which of these types of events is most likely to occur and why?

References

1. Centers for Disease Control and Prevention. Chemical categories. *Emergency Preparedness and Response.* Available at http://emergency.cdc.gov/agent/agentlistchem-category.asp. Updated April 8, 2013. Accessed March 1, 2015.
2. Centers for Disease Control and Prevention. Chemical emergencies overview. *Emergency Preparedness and Response.* Available at http://emergency.cdc.gov/chemical/overview.asp. Updated April 17, 2013. Accessed February 6, 2016.
3. Centers for Disease Control and Prevention. Facts about Sulfur Mustard. *Emergency Preparedness and Response.* Available at http://emergency.cdc.gov/agent/sulfurmustard/basics/facts.asp. Updated May 2, 2013. Accessed March 8, 2015.
4. Centers for Disease Control and Prevention. Facts about Lewisite. *Emergency Preparedness and Response.* Available at http://emergency.cdc.gov/agent/lewisite/basics/facts.asp. Updated March 14, 2013. Accessed March 8, 2015.
5. Agency for Toxic Substances and Disease Registry. Toxic substances portal—Sulfur Mustard. ToxFAQs™ for Sulfur Mustard. Available at http://www.atsdr.cdc.gov/toxfaqs/tf.asp?id=904&tid=184. Updated June 27, 2013. Accessed March 8, 2015.
6. Katz R. *Essentials of Public Health Preparedness.* Burlington, MA: Jones & Bartlett Learning; 2013.
7. Yourish K, Rebecca Lai KK, Watkins D. Deaths in Syria. *New York Times.* Available at http://www.nytimes.com/interactive/2015/09/14/world/middleeast/syria-war-deaths.html. Published September 14, 2015. Accessed October 11, 2015.
8. Chivers CJ. What an ISIS chemical strike did to one Syrian family. *New York Times.* October 6, 2015. Available at http://www.nytimes.com/2015/10/07/world/middleeast/syrian-familys-agony-raises-specter-of-chemical-warfare.html?_r=0. Accessed October 11, 2015.
9. Centers for Disease Control and Prevention. Facts about Cyanide. *Emergency Preparedness and Response.* Available at http://emergency.cdc.gov/agent/cyanide/basics/facts.asp. Updated June 27, 2013. Accessed July 15, 2015.
10. 1988: Thousands die in Halabja gas attack. *BBCNews. On This Day.* Available at http://news.bbc.co.uk/onthisday/hi/dates/stories/march/16/newsid_4304000/4304853. March 16, 1988. Accessed July 17, 2015.
11. Centers for Disease Control and Prevention. Facts about Chlorine. *Emergency Preparedness and Response.* Available at http://emergency.cdc.gov/agent/chlorine/basics/facts.asp. Updated April 10, 2013. Accessed July 17, 2015.
12. Centers for Disease Control and Prevention. Facts about Phosgene. *Emergency Preparedness and Response.* Available at http://emergency.cdc.gov/agent/phosgene/basics/facts.asp. Updated April 12, 2013. Accessed July 17, 2015.
13. Choking agents. Organisation for the Prohibition of Chemical Weapons. Available at https://www.opcw.org/protection/types-of-Chemical-Agent/Choking-Agents/. Accessed October 11, 2015.
14. Limaye Y. Bhopal chemical leak site 30 years on. *BBC News.* Available at http://www.bbc.com/news/world-asia-30301659. December 3, 2014. Accessed October 11, 2015.
15. Matiash C. 30 years later, suffering continues in Bhopal. *Wall Street Journal.* Available at http://www.wsj.com/articles/photos-30-years-later-suffering-continues-in-bhopal-1417644275. December 3, 2014. Accessed October 11, 2015.
16. Centers for Disease Control and Prevention. Facts about Sarin. *Emergency Preparedness and Response.* Available at http://emergency.cdc.gov/agent/sarin/basics/facts.asp. Updated May 20, 2013. Accessed October 18, 2015.

17. Centers for Disease Control and Prevention. Facts about Tabun. *Emergency Preparedness and Response.* Available at http://emergency.cdc.gov/agent/tabun/basics/facts.asp. Updated March 27, 2013. Accessed October 18, 2015.

18. Lindsay, JM. Lessons learned: Tokyo Sarin gas attack. Council on foreign relations. Video. Available at http://www.cfr.org/japan/lessons-learned-tokyo-sarin-gas-attack/p27685. Published March 20, 2012. Accessed November 15, 2015.

19. CDC. CDC's CHEMPACK Program—The Stockpile that may protect you from a chemical attack. *Public Health Matters Blog.* Available at http://blogs.cdc.gov/publichealthmatters/2015/02/cdcs-chempack-program-the-stockpile-that-may-protect-you-from-a-chemical-attack/. Published February 19, 2015. Accessed November 15, 2015.

20. Harvard PERLC/PERRC and Massachusetts Department of Public Health. Del Valle Institute for Emergency Preparedness Learning Center. Massachusetts CHEMPACK Training Program. 3 Modules. Available at https://delvalle.bphc.org/course/view.php?id=361. Published February 2011. Accessed May 7, 2014; November 29, 2015.

21. Organisation for the Prohibition of Chemical Weapons. Chemical Weapons Convention. Available at https://www.opcw.org/chemical-weapons-convention/. Accessed February 7, 2016.

22. Centers for Disease Control and Prevention. Bioterrorism overview. *Emergency Preparedness and Response.* Available at http://emergency.cdc.gov/bioterrorism/overview.asp. Updated February 12, 2007. Accessed February 7, 2016.

23. Nicolson, G. Emergency response disaster management. *Bioterrorism and Biological Warfare Agents.* Available at http://www.immed.org/illness/bioterrorism.html. Published 2001. Accessed February 11, 2016.

24. Gilad J, Harary I, Dushnitsky T, Schwartz D. *Burkholderia Mallei* and *Burkholderia Pseudomallei* as bioterrorism agents: a national aspects of emergency preparedness. *Israeli Med Assoc J.* 2007;9:499–503. Available at http://www.ima.org.il/FilesUpload/IMAJ/0/46/23087.pdf. Accessed February 13, 2016.

25. Centers for Disease Control and Prevention. Biological and chemical terrorism: strategic plan for preparedness and response. *MMWR.* 2000;49:1–26. Available at http://www.cdc.gov/mmwr/pdf/rr/rr4904.pdf. Accessed February 13, 2016.

26. International Atomic Energy Agency. What is a radiological emergency? Available at http://www-ns.iaea.org/tech-areas/emergency/iec/frg/what-is-a-rad-emergency.asp. Accessed August 31, 2017.

27. U.S. Department of Homeland Security. Nuclear blast. Available at https://www.ready.gov/nuclear-blast. Accessed August 31, 2017.

28. Federation of American Scientists. Nuclear & radiological terrorism. Available at https://fas.org/issues/nuclear-and-radiological-terrorism/. Accessed August 31, 2017.

29. Bulletin of the Atomic Scientists. What does nuclear terrorism really mean? Available at http://thebulletin.org/what-does-nuclear-terrorism-really-mean9309. Accessed August 31, 2017.

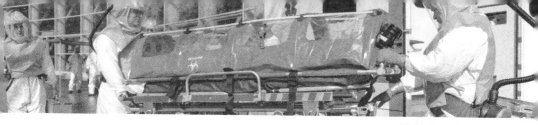

CHAPTER 4

Natural Disasters and Unintentional Emergencies

LEARNING OBJECTIVES

The public health emergencies that generate the most fear and media coverage may be human-caused events, such as terrorist attacks, but every year the number of people affected by natural disasters is far greater than the number of people affected by terrorist attacks. Even when natural disasters are not widespread and devastating to millions, the total of an average year's storms, floods, mudslides, blizzards, naturally caused forest fires, tornados, and power outages affects millions of Americans.

In many cases, natural disasters can be predicted and planned for to some degree. Communities in Tornado Alley have a reasonable expectation of tornados each spring and summer. The San Francisco Bay Area has been preparing for a major earthquake for decades. The East Coast routinely gets practice responding to winter weather events, and Gulf Coast states know that hurricane season brings a threat every year. But even with extensive planning, training, and drilling, the magnitude of natural disasters can stretch response capabilities to their limit.

By the end of this chapter, readers should be able to:

- Understand the various types of natural disasters and their impacts on public health
- Understand special concerns with regard to the various types of natural disasters
- Identify and define unintentional emergencies
- Articulate potential public health impacts of unintentional emergencies

▶ Natural Disasters

Introduction

Humans recall natural disasters vividly. Images of destruction, devastation, and loss are etched in our brains from recent occurrences of natural disasters, most recently from Hurricane/Tropical Storm Harvey that made landfall on August 25, 2017, in Texas. After a devastating natural disaster, such as a hurricane or flood, assistance comes from governments, nongovernmental organizations, and others in the form of humanitarian relief, search and rescue operations, cleanup, and rebuilding. The toll on humans is often significant. The magnitude of natural disasters often challenges response efforts, and the scale of their impact may even highlight gaps in planning and resources.

For every natural disaster humans remember, there are countless others we do not. Wildfires, floods, tornadoes, hurricanes, and blizzards occur annually in the United States. In 2015 and 2016, wildfires and flooding in South Carolina, Texas, Oklahoma, and Louisiana made headlines in the media and faded as the next incident occurred.

While natural disasters can be predicted, planning for their full impact can be somewhat elusive. Natural disasters are unpreventable, often unpredictable incidents whose onset can be acute or gradual. Also, natural disasters cannot be confined to a geographical area, so planning for response to these types of disasters can be significant, especially in areas that are prone to frequent occurrence of these disasters. Maintaining knowledge of natural threats and their impacts can help communities plan mitigation/prevention, response, and recovery efforts.

As with all other emergencies, building relationships across all levels of government and throughout communities is essential to developing deep-rooted community resilience that can contribute significantly to community recovery. Forecasters can use sophisticated technology to predict severe weather and issue warnings to potentially affected areas. Wildfires, flooding, or hurricanes may require evacuation. Disasters often adversely affect the most vulnerable populations in an area. Although public health organizations and individuals are experts in disaster planning and response, missteps with dire consequences do happen. These missteps often relate to the intricacies of timing and communication.

Again, natural disasters can be acute or gradual. Natural disasters with acute onsets include

- Earthquakes
- Floods
- Hurricanes and typhoons
- Tornados
- Tsunamis
- Storm surges
- Others: avalanches, volcanic eruptions, extreme weather (cold, heat, blizzards)

Those with more gradual onset include droughts, famine, desertification, and deforestation.[1] As depicted in **TABLE 4-1**, natural disasters can have significant environmental impacts. These environmental effects can cause a number of public health challenges during mitigation.

Potential Public Health Impacts

Slow-moving, often escapable natural disasters, such as hurricanes, wildfires, and floods, tend to have lower rates of death and injury in the immediate aftermath. Conversely, the more acute events, including earthquakes and tornados, tend to cause higher rates of death and injury in the immediate aftermath. Following are some of the potential public health concerns that may affect an emergency response across many different types of natural disasters:

TABLE 4-1 Natural Disasters and Their Environmental Impact

Natural Disaster	Environmental Effects
Blizzard/coldwave/ heavy snowfall	Avalanche, erosion, snow melt (flooding), loss of plants and animals, river ice jams (flooding)
Cyclone	Flooding, landslide, erosion, loss of plant and animal life
Drought	Fire, depletion of water resources, deterioration of soil, loss of plant and animal life
Earthquake	Landslide, rock fall, avalanche
Flood/thunderstorm	Heavy rainfall, fire, landslide, erosion, destruction of plant life
Heat wave	Fire, loss of plants and animals, depletion of water resources, deterioration of soil, snow melt (flooding)
Lightning	Fire
Thunderstorm/heavy rainfall	Flooding, fire, landslide, erosion, destruction of plant life
Tornado	Loss of plant and animal life, erosion, water disturbance
Tsunami	Flooding, erosion, loss of plant and animal life
Volcanic eruption	Loss of plant and animal life, deterioration of soil, air and water pollution
Wildfires	Destruction of ground cover, erosion, flooding, mudslides, long-term smog, and tainted soil

Data from American Public Health Association. Types of Disasters and Their Consequences. Available at: www.medscape.com /viewarticle/513258_2. Accessed August 20, 2017.

- Displacement of people
- Sanitation in crowded living conditions
- Water supply contamination
- Damage to healthcare infrastructure
- Mental health impacts
- Nutrition and food availability
- Communicable disease
- Availability of medications to treat chronic illnesses
- Exposure (to extreme heat or cold)
- Power outages
- Damage to public infrastructure such as transportation systems and roadways
- Vulnerable populations who may be trapped

Some natural disasters entail additional threats and special concerns that must also be addressed in disaster response plans. Floods, hurricanes, earthquakes, and extreme weather events especially require careful planning to ensure robust responses. As is often seen, these disasters in particular can lead to other compounding issues that have the potential for magnifying the response and creating additional public health challenges that will also need to be mitigated.

Special Concerns in Floods and Hurricanes

All around the world, flooding is the most common type of disaster, and in the United States, flash floods are the leading cause of weather-related deaths. Climate change and more frequently alternating ocean oscillations mean that hurricanes of Category 3 or greater now hit the continental United States approximately every 18 months, often bringing devastating floods.[2]

Water pipes and sewage systems can quickly become overwhelmed during flood events, leading to contamination of drinking systems and the "toxic soup" of flood water, sewage, gasoline, and chemicals through which we often see survivors wade in news footage. For survivors and rescuers alike, flood waters pose a deceptive threat: what looks like regular rainwater is actually full of bacteria and toxins that can accidentally be ingested or absorbed through even the smallest cuts or abrasions on the skin. In the months after a flood, stagnant water can also become a breeding ground for mosquitoes, which are vectors for diseases such as Zika and West Nile Virus.

When the flood waters recede, communities and individuals will find themselves in a race against mold. Mold is common in post-flood locations and can pose a serious threat to the public's health. Experts generally recommend that anything touched by flood water be removed and replaced, including drywall and carpeting. Because this is such a costly and time-consuming effort, those in lower socioeconomic communities may not be able to afford to remove mold and rebuild homes and places of business, leading to a secondary and slow-moving public health disaster that unfolds over years.

Response efforts during massive flooding may be complicated by the inability to drive emergency vehicles on submerged roads. When responders are required to travel by boat or helicopter, a response effort can be greatly slowed. While floods cause the greatest number of deaths, most people are able to heed weather reports and evacuation warnings to avoid affected areas and stay out of harm. Despite an effective communication campaign, there will always be those who refuse evacuation orders. Establishing trusted agents within the community will help emergency planners ensure that bridges are created to fill perceived gaps between emergency responders and citizens. In flash floods, which can develop very quickly, anticipated rainfall events often provide enough warning to alert those living or traveling in flash flood zones. But even when floods do not cause deaths, they can leave large numbers of displaced survivors in their wake. Public health professionals must select shelter sites and plan for their operation, taking into account such considerations as food preparation, sanitary conditions, medications and other supplies, water availability, and accessibility to those with disabilities. Because certain communities or demographic groups may not heed government messages, trusted agents will be able to communicate these messages more effectively within communities and across demographic groups. We discuss this further in Chapter 11.

Special Concerns in Earthquakes

Major earthquakes are relatively rare in the United States, but it takes only one to cause a massive public health disaster that will affect a community for years. However, minor earthquakes have been occurring in the United States at an alarmingly higher rate in the last several years. According to the U.S. Geological Survey (USGS), "between the years 1973 and 2008, there was an average of 21 earthquakes of magnitude 3 and larger in the central and eastern United States,"[3] but this rate has ballooned to more than 600 earthquakes of magnitude 3 or larger in 2014 and over 1000 in 2015 alone.[3] USGS scientists are currently studying this increased seismic activity, which is believed to be induced by human behavior due to practices like underground wastewater injection for fracking. Regardless, earthquakes remain a serious threat to areas along fault lines and are a growing threat to areas that previously were unaffected. Today, "more than 143 million Americans live in areas of significant seismic risk across 39 states."[4] "In the next 30 years, California has a 99.7% chance of a magnitude 6.7 or larger earthquake and the Pacific Northwest has a 10% chance of a magnitude 8–9 megathrust earthquake on the Cascadia subduction zone."[4]

Earthquakes strike with little or no warning, so there is no chance for people in an affected zone to evacuate. For this reason, earthquakes tend to have a higher rate of injury and death in the immediate aftermath. Most casualties are caused by collapsing buildings due to ground displacement and soil liquefaction, but earthquakes often come with secondary threats, such as widespread fires and damage to nuclear facilities, that can be even more damaging than the earthquakes themselves.

Fires can be a particularly dangerous hazard following an earthquake. Ruptured gas lines and arcing electrical wires are the most common sources of ignition,[5] and obstructed roadways and damaged water supply systems can make it difficult for firefighters to access sites. For example, after the 1995 earthquake in Kobe, Japan, fire combined with the effects of the earthquake resulted in the destruction of 150,000 buildings when water supplies were depleted and water tankers could not reach their destinations.[6]

Exposure and poor air quality are significant hazards following an earthquake. Because earthquakes can happen at any time of year, exposure may become a threat for displaced survivors and those who have intact homes but lack electricity. This problem becomes particularly dangerous for vulnerable populations such as the elderly and the homebound. Soil liquefaction results in the collapse of buildings that releases particulate matter into the air. As a result, air quality can be poor immediately after an earthquake and pose a threat for the very young, the very old, and those with compromised immune systems or respiratory conditions.

The USGS is working to develop early warning systems that may be able to alert communities and individuals to earthquakes before the shaking reaches them. While these systems would provide only seconds or tens of seconds of warning, those precious seconds could enable trains and taxiing planes to stop, workers to move away from dangerous machines or chemicals, students to take cover under desks, and power plants and industrial systems to shut down.[4] These mitigation tactics can significantly decrease injuries and deaths as well as secondary threats such as fires.

Special Concerns in Extreme Temperatures

In extreme temperatures, exposure due to heat or cold is a problem disproportionately experienced by vulnerable communities, such as the elderly or chronically ill. Residents may lack the resources to pay for gas or electricity to power a furnace during the winter or lack a climate-controlled shelter in the summer. The adverse effects of heat waves and extreme cold are largely preventable with careful planning that includes early warning systems, timely public notification and medical advice, improvements at the housing and urban planning level, and partnerships with social systems and community organizations.[7]

It should also be noted that during heat waves, power grids can be overwhelmed by heavy use and cause widespread power outages. In these situations, heat exposure can rapidly become a threat to a much larger population. Socio-economic factors can further increase risk for injury or death during times of extreme temperatures. The 1995 heat wave in Chicago, IL demonstrated how socio-economic factors can significantly increase risks during disasters. In that event, over 700 people died as a result of exposure to extreme heat. A large portion of those were poor, elderly and socially isolated individuals living in poor communities with high crime rates. Out of fear for their safety and to guard against break-ins, many of these residents remained in their non-air-conditioned homes, windows shut, essentially baking to death. In his book "Heat Wave: A Social Autopsy of Disaster in Chicago," Eric Klinenberg details the effects the weeklong heat wave had on the city and its most vulnerable residents.[8]

▶ Unintentional Emergencies

Introduction

In emergency preparedness, a final category of hazards and threats encompasses all unintentional emergencies. Unintentional emergencies are, in essence, unplanned accidents. They can include

- Power outages
- Hazardous materials spills
- Train derailments
- Foodborne outbreaks

While public health would not be the lead agency in a power outage, hazardous materials spill, or train derailment, it is the lead agency during a foodborne outbreak. As a result, core leadership, management, communication, and planning principles and skills are inherent in public health practice, and public health would be a strong collaborative partner during an unintentional emergency. Public health would also be responsible for bringing nontraditional responders into the response effort during any of these emergencies. For example, in an evacuation scenario involving persons who take multiple medications but evacuate without them may necessitate partnering with a local pharmacy to provide prescription refills to evacuees. In this type of scenario, public health officials would be responsible for coordinating this service with a pharmacy provider and setting up the temporary pharmacy for services to be provided.

Special Concerns in Power Outages

Power outages have many causes, from weather related to accidental, and they have the potential for significant impacts on public health because countless public services cannot be delivered without electricity. For example, in the 2003 New York City blackout, water pumps that relied on electricity were unable to operate. Public health officials issued a water boil advisory, but the means to communicate it to the public also relied on electricity. Finally, many residents could not follow a boil order anyway because electric stoves and microwaves would not function. As this example illustrates, a power outage can have a domino effect.[9]

Because power outages lead to an increased use of generators, these events often cause a spike in carbon monoxide exposures. One study found that the most common cause of disaster-related carbon monoxide poisoning was generator use, which was attributed to 54% of nonfatal cases and 83% of fatal cases.[9,10]

Evacuation may even be necessary in a seemingly nonurgent incident such as a power outage that affects a healthcare facility or a residential high-rise building in which elevators no longer function. Large-scale evacuations can require the capability to relocate those who are displaced, either to alternate housing, housing with family members, or perhaps to emergency shelters. In the case of emergency shelters, other needs of the displaced may have to be accommodated, including feeding, sanitation, medication (for those who evacuate without prescription medications), and care of personal pets.[11]

Special Concerns in Hazardous Materials Spills

Hazardous materials (hazmat) spills can have a wide range of impacts on a community depending on the type of material spilled (oil, ammonia, gasoline, corrosives, radioactive materials, explosives, and other material), the location in which it was spilled (residential versus rural), and the quantity. Interventions can include decontamination, shelter-in-place, evacuation, and restricting access to the affected area. In the case of hazardous chemical releases that can be harmful to the public's health, many of the plans and approaches will be similar to those used in the case of an intentional chemical release, such as a terrorist attack, which include near-immediate medical care and the provision of medical countermeasures.

Special Concerns in Train Derailments

Train derailments can cause a variety of effects, largely depending on what the train was carrying. Passenger trains will require a heavy medical response, while freight train derailments could—in worst-case scenarios—require a hazmat response. For example, the train derailment on July 6, 2013, in Canada resulted in a fire and explosions in the town of Lac-Mégantic. Seventy-two train cars filled with crude oil raced toward the town when the brake system failed. Forty-seven people were killed, while 2000 had to be evacuated in the early morning hours. The investigation revealed that gaps in safety and human error were to blame, and the incident prompted action both in Canada and the United States to tighten regulations for the tank car involved as well as to ensure additional safety protections in populated areas.[12]

Special Concerns in Foodborne Outbreaks

Unintentional emergencies can also cause a large degree of illness. In 2011, a multi-state outbreak of listeriosis infections was traced to whole cantaloupes from a farm in Colorado.[13] A total of 147 people were infected across 28 states, and 33 died. In these incidents, the work of epidemiologists is critical to determining the cause.

More localized incidents of foodborne illness can stress local health systems. For example, in 2007 at the Taste of Chicago, the city's annual outdoor food festival, contaminated hummus sickened up to 770 people. Of those, 158 cases tested positive as salmonella. By interviewing affected people, the Chicago Department of Public Health determined that all of those affected had visited the same food stand at the festival. Dozens were hospitalized with symptoms of salmonella poisoning, putting added stress on the local health system.[14] In larger, perhaps multistate foodborne outbreaks, the stress to healthcare systems can be far more severe. In a multistate foodborne outbreak, the U.S. Centers for Disease Control will take the lead role in the response. These outbreak investigations have three goals, which include:

1. "Quickly detect outbreaks
2. Gather the evidence
3. Communicate to consumers and retailers about the source of the outbreak"[15]

A strong surveillance and epidemiology infrastructure is key to the emergency response to foodborne outbreaks.

▶ Conclusion

Natural disasters affect more persons per year than any other type of disaster. Natural disasters can also cause widespread damage and destruction, often leaving communities completely decimated. Because of the catastrophic destruction caused by some natural disasters, recovery efforts may be long-term, expensive endeavors. Preparedness for natural disasters must include additional considerations, including how to care for the social needs of the displaced, as well as the healthcare needs. As such, emergency planners must understand the special concerns associated with various types of natural disasters, as well as the cascading effects they can have.

In all emergencies, including those that are unintentional, the public health infrastructure is key to the quality of the emergency response. Planning for the unexpected can be difficult, but by building flexibility and scalability into preparedness plans, public health practitioners can mitigate their effects on healthcare systems and the public at large.

Discussion Questions

1. Name three acute natural disasters. What are the special concerns with each of these types of disasters?
2. What are some of the additional hazards that can be caused by a catastrophic-level flood?
3. What are unintentional emergencies?
4. Why are unintentional emergencies of great concern to public health?

References

1. American Public Health Association. Types of disasters and their consequences. Available at http://www.medscape.com/viewarticle/513258_2. Accessed August 20, 2017.
2. Diaz JH. The public health impact of hurricanes and major flooding. *J Louisiana State Med Soc: Off Organ Louisiana State Med Soc.* 2004;156(3):145–150.
3. United States Geological Survey. Induced earthquakes. Available at https://earthquake.usgs.gov/research/induced/. Accessed August 20, 2017.
4. Shake Alert. Shake Alert: Earthquake early warning. Available at https://www.shakealert.org/. Accessed August 20, 2017.
5. Pacific Northwest Seismic Network. Fire. Available at https://pnsn.org/outreach/earthquakehazards/fire. Accessed August 24, 2017.
6. National Institute of Standards and Technology. Earthquake Kobe Japan 1995. Available at https://www.nist.gov/el/earthquake-kobe-japan-1995. Accessed August 30, 2017.
7. World Health Organization. Heat-health action plans. Available at http://www.euro.who.int/__data/assets/pdf_file/0006/95919/E91347.pdf?ua=1. Accessed August 24, 2017.
8. Klinenberg, E. *Heat Wave: A Social Autopsy of Disaster in Chicago.* Chicago, IL: University of Chicago Press; 2002.
9. Klinger C, Landeg O, Murray V. Power outages, extreme events and health: a systematic review of the literature from 2011–2012. *PLOS Currents Disaster.* Published January 2, 2014. doi:10.1371/currents.dis.04eb1dc5e73dd1377e05a10e9edde673.
10. Centers for Disease Control and Prevention. Notes from the field: carbon monoxide exposures reported to poison centers and related to Hurricane Sandy – Northeastern United States, 2012 *MMWR.* November 9, 2012;61(44):905.
11. Thompson K, Every D, Rainbird S, Cornell V, Smith B, Trigg J. No pet or their person left behind: increasing the disaster resilience of Vulnerable Groups through animal attachment, activities and networks. *Animals : An Open Access Journal from MDPI.* 2014;4(2):214–240. doi:10.3390/ani4020214.
12. Halsey A. Canadian runaway oil train disaster blamed on 'weak safety culture,' poor oversight. *The Washington Post.* The Americas. Available at https://www.washingtonpost.com/world/the_americas/canadian-runaway-train-disaster-blamed-on-weak-safety-culture-poor-oversight/2014/08/19/8ac42280-27b5-11e4-8593-da634b334390_story.html?utm_term=.6388dd708b8f. Published August 19, 2014. Accessed September 2, 2017.
13. U.S. Centers for Disease Control and Prevention. Multistate outbreak of listeriosis linked to whole cantaloupes from Jensen Farms, Colorado (FINAL UPDATE). Available at https://www.cdc.gov/listeria/outbreaks/cantaloupes-jensen-farms/index.html. Accessed August 30, 2017.
14. Food Poison Journal. Salmonella outbreak at Taste of Chicago. Available at http://www.foodpoisonjournal.com/foodborne-illness-outbreaks/salmonella-outbreak-at-taste-of-chicago/. Published July 12, 2007. Accessed August 30, 2017.
15. Centers for Disease Control and Prevention. CDC's role during investigations of multistate outbreaks linked to food or animal contact. Available at https://www.cdc.gov/foodsafety/outbreaks/multistate-outbreaks/cdc-role.html. Updated August 16, 2016. Accessed August 30, 2017.

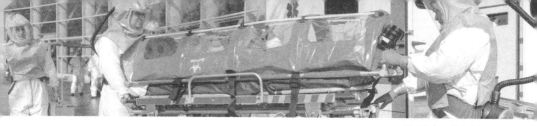

CHAPTER 5
Pandemic Influenza

LEARNING OBJECTIVES

One of the greatest threats to the public's health today is the threat of a novel strain of influenza, with a high degree of pandemic potential. There were three occurrences of pandemic influenza in the 20th century: the 1918–1919 Spanish flu, the 1957–1958 Asian flu, and the 1968–1969 Hong Kong flu. The worst of these three, the 1918–1919 Spanish flu, spread rapidly around the world, killing over 20 million people worldwide.

The ease and quick nature of international travel has brought great cause and concern to public health officials in the United States, as international travel dramatically increases the likelihood that a novel strain of flu or other infectious disease could be introduced into the country with little to no notice. This concern was heightened in the early part of the 21st century with the spread of a highly pathogenic strain of avian influenza (H5N1) that spread from Asia to Europe and Africa.[1] As a result, emergency planners in the United States began planning for the possibility of H5N1 to be introduced into the country. To date, the United States has not experienced a strain of influenza as virulent as that of the Spanish flu of 1918, nor H5N1; however, the 2009–2010 H1N1 pandemic served as a reminder to emergency planners that a highly pathogenic strain of a novel influenza continues to be a great threat to the public's health.

By the end of this chapter, readers should be able to:

- Understand how global disease poses a threat to the nation's health security
- Define pandemic influenza
- Distinguish the differences between seasonal influenza and pandemic influenza
- Understand the emergency response elements necessary to mitigate the effects of emerging and reemerging infectious disease outbreaks

▶ Health Security

What is health security? Health security is "a state in which the nation and its people are prepared for, protected from and resilient in the face of health threats or incidents with potentially negative health consequences."[2(p33)] The National Health Security Strategy (NHSS) was released in December 2009 and focused on a "whole community" approach to preparedness and response to emergency events. The goals of the strategy include protecting the public's health during an emergency and guiding the nation's efforts to minimize the risks associated with a wide range of potential large-scale incidents that put the health and well-being of the nation's people at risk.

Global Disease as a Threat

The emergence of a myriad of diseases has caused infectious diseases to become recognized as a threat to the nation's security. Examples of such diseases include the HIV/AIDS epidemic, Ebola, cholera, drug-resistant tuberculosis, severe acute respiratory syndrome, and H1N1. As indicated in the NHSS, "the threat of contagious diseases transcends political boundaries, and the ability to prevent, quickly detect and contain outbreaks with pandemic potential has never been so important."[2(p36)]

Global interconnectedness, aided by the ease of international travel, has heightened the concern of potential pandemics and their impact. This interconnectedness has also made the United States more susceptible to the introduction of exotic, uncommon infectious diseases that the U.S. public health and healthcare system have not had to confront previously. The emergence of previously unseen, and sometime highly pathogenic, infectious diseases creates a specific challenge in that hospitals, healthcare systems, and public health systems may not have the resources and treatment interventions necessary to readily mitigate the newly emerging threat. As was seen during the Ebola outbreak in 2014, specialized equipment and training were needed not only to care for potentially affected patients but also to ensure the protection of healthcare workers responsible for providing patient care. Effective isolation, patient assessment, diagnosis, and treatment required designated treatment rooms and equipment, resulting in the removal of these resources from daily, routine use within facilities designated to care for potentially infected patients, or patients under investigation for Ebola infection. Newly emerging infectious diseases put the United States at risk of shortages in healthcare personnel and medical supplies needed for proper patient care. Traditional medical school curricula do not include courses or seminars that teach future physicians how to recognize the symptoms of and be able to diagnose exotic infectious diseases or illness resulting from other biological agents, which further burdens public health epidemiological and surveillance experts in tracking and identifying the definition of and source of infection. Thus, it is increasingly important for broad participation and collaboration among public health systems, healthcare systems, and other public safety partners to ensure timely and effective identification of disease agents and proper treatment and other response efforts.[3]

Global Surveillance

Global disease threats require diligent surveillance activities to protect countries from large-scale emerging and reemerging infectious disease outbreaks. Several outbreaks over the last decade of the 20th century demonstrated the consequences that delayed national recognition and response to outbreaks could have. Those consequences include illness and death of national populations including health workers, potential spread to other countries, and significant disruptions in travel and trade, thus adversely affecting the economic viability of countries.[4] Surveillance is the hallmark of public health response, and inadequate surveillance and response capability in one area of the world can endanger national populations and the public health security of the entire world.[4] During emergencies, public health officials need to ensure the availability of epidemiology and disease surveillance tools and systems, including the capability to identify disease incidence, disease prevalence, and severity of illness. Epidemiology and surveillance staff need to have the capacity to quickly process, analyze, and interpret data. Data are integral to decision-making during an emergency. Data may come from a variety of sources including syndromic surveillance mechanisms, such as community medical providers, hospital emergency departments and healthcare systems, sentinel surveillance systems, and other data reporting systems. Epidemiology activities include conducting epidemiological investigations, determining exposure risk, identifying populations in need of prophylaxis, providing recommendations to the healthcare community and public, determining criteria to be used for identification of cases and controls, and monitoring morbidity and mortality associated with the emergency.[5(p94)]

Etiology of Influenza Viruses

Influenza is a respiratory illness characterized by fever, headache, tiredness, dry cough, sore throat, runny nose, muscle aches, and occasionally nausea, vomiting, and diarrhea. Complications occur mostly among high-risk individuals and include bacterial pneumonia, dehydration, and worsening of chronic conditions such as congestive heart disease, asthma, and diabetes.[6,7] Flu strains are typically found in mammals. Birds and swine are the most common hosts for what typically become human flu viruses. Flu viruses thrive in the winter but virtually disappear in the summer. This is because flu viruses "move" to the cold side of the planet for survival. Flu hosts usually develop an immunity to the virus after infection. Flu survives by overcoming seasonal influences and mutating to change the immunity in its target population. It is widely accepted that individuals who routinely get an annual flu vaccine typically have a higher resistance to emerging flu strains than those who do not.

Some segments of the human population can be at higher risk for influenza infection. Thus, diligence and careful treatment are imperative for these groups of individuals. High-risk individuals include those who are over the age of 65 or under the age of 2, as well as those with chronic illnesses. Persons with HIV, lymphomas, and other immune-compromising conditions are also at increased risk. Influenza infectivity is relatively high, with a short incubation period, generally lasting 2–3 days for most flus. Clinical illness is also nonspecific in that it looks like many other illnesses, with symptoms such as headache, slight fever, and muscle aches. Influenza is also easily transmitted. As shown in **FIGURE 5-1**, flu is most commonly transmitted through large, airborne droplets from coughing, sneezing, or contact with saliva. A more rare form of transmission is airborne travel over long distances. "The average impact of influenza is infection of about 5% to 20% of the population.

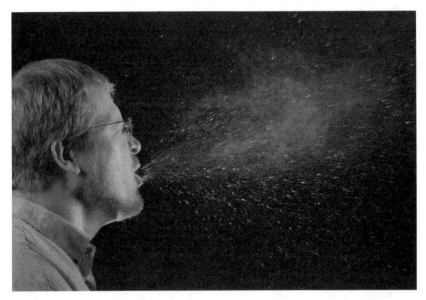

FIGURE 5-1 Airborne droplets from sneezing
Courtesy of CDC/Brian Judd/James Gathany.

Typically, over 200,000 people in the U.S. are hospitalized annually. In about half of these hospitalizations, those affected are persons over the age of 65. Annually, the average death rate from influenza in the U.S. is 36,000 deaths per year with more than 90% of these deaths occurring in persons over the age of 65."[7] These numbers do not typically tax hospitals and emergency rooms; however, a larger number of infections from pandemic strains of flu could tax the U.S. healthcare system.

Figure 5-1 illustrates a very effective way to spread the disease. Similar to the admonishment that your mother gave you about covering your cough or sneeze and washing your hands after, good respiratory hygiene is still the best protection against flu infection. This is because most changes in influenza viruses from one year to the next are minor changes or mutations. This is why those who routinely get an annual flu vaccine typically have a higher resistance to the next year's flu strains, or even emerging flu strains, than those who do not. Small mutations in the viral structure are called *antigenic drifts*. When a flu virus drifts slightly, the vaccine may be close enough to cover the drift and thus protect the individual from that particular strain of flu. However, when flu viruses change significantly, an *antigenic shift* occurs. This is a more significant change, and the vaccine may not provide full protection of the strain. If researchers can predict the shift, it is possible to change the flu vaccine in order to cover the new virus (**FIGURE 5-2**). Also, when there is a major antigenic shift in the immunologic structure, it generally results in a pandemic.[8]

Pandemic Influenza

A pandemic strain of influenza occurs about every 50–70 years. Influenza pandemics spread over a wide geographic area, typically worldwide. Pandemic strains usually affect a high percentage of the population because most people do not have

Influenza: antigenic drift and shift

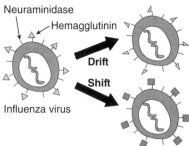

FIGURE 5-2 Antigenic drift versus shift

Data from A Train Education: Continuing Education for Healthcare Professionals. Available at: www.atrainceu.com/course-all
/influenza-familiar-but-deadly-133. Accessed: April 4, 2017.

protection from the new or "novel" strain, and no vaccine is available. As a result, pandemic strains tend to have higher disease attack rates and higher death rates than seasonal or normal influenza.

In the 20th century, three influenza pandemics occurred around the world. The Hong Kong flu occurred in 1968–1969. The mildest of the three pandemics, the Hong Kong flu caused 34,000 deaths in the United States, about the same number that the United States continues to see annually from seasonal flu. By these standards, the Hong Kong flu would be considered mild and not of "pandemic proportion." In 1957, the Asian flu killed 70,000 people in the United States, about double the rate of seasonal influenza deaths in the United States.[7]

By far, the worst and most deadly of these three pandemics was the Spanish flu, which occurred in 1918–1919. Characterized by widespread illness and death, the 1918 pandemic caused 20 million deaths worldwide, and more than 650,000 in the United States.[7] To date, the 1918 Spanish flu remains on record as the deadliest strain of influenza to ever occur in the United States and the world.[9]

When pandemics spread, they spread rapidly around the world in repeating waves. In 1918, the wave circled the globe in 6–9 months. This pandemic also had a high death rate among young adults. About one in every 100 young adults, aged 25–34 years, died during the 1918 pandemic. This is a lesson that pandemic flu can behave very differently than seasonal flu. In 1918, the groups most at risk were not the old or necessarily the infirm, as peaks for the deaths were all under the age of 50. See **FIGURES 5-3** and **5-4**.

Impact of Pandemic Influenza

Pandemic influenza is extremely disruptive to societies, their functioning, and the economy. Typically, in pandemic situations, we see large rates of worker absenteeism and lost productivity due to the inability to obtain or transport supplies and raw materials. We also see disruptions in utilities and critical infrastructure, as the ability to access fuel and basic utilities, telecommunications, and information technology systems is uncertain. The availability of public safety personnel and public services as well as food and medical suppliers is affected. Pandemics also bring increased demands on the healthcare infrastructure and the workforce. From an economic perspective, reduced tourism, travel, entertaining, and the hospitality industries can

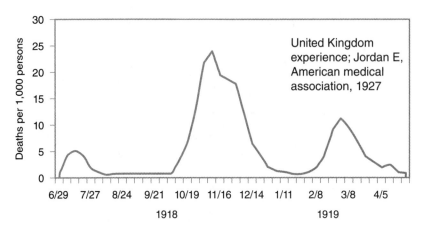

FIGURE 5-3 1918 Pandemic waves

Data from Taubenberger JK, Morens DM. 1918 Influenza: the Mother of All Pandemics. Emerging Infectious Diseases. 2006;12(1): 15-22. Jordan, E. Epidemic Influenza: A Survey. Chicago: American Medical Association, 1927. Available at: www.nc.cdc.gov/eid /article/12/1/05-0979_article. Accessed April 4, 2017.

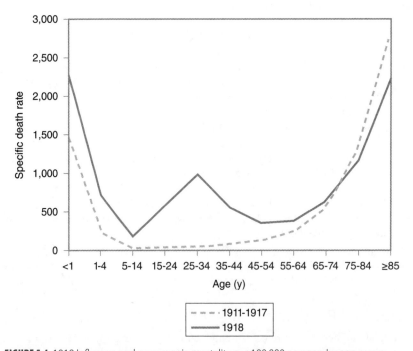

FIGURE 5-4 1918 Influenza and pneumonia mortality per 100,000 persons, by age group

Data from Taubenberger JK, Morens DM. 1918 Influenza: the Mother of All Pandemics. Emerging Infectious Diseases. 2006;12(1):15-22. Available at: www.nc.cdc.gov/eid/article/12/1/05-0979_article Accessed: April 4, 2017.

be negatively affected, due to low rates of occupancy and tourism. Because pandemic effects are widespread, there is no help available from other areas, as they are also affected. This is why pandemic influenza planning and preparedness is so critical for emergency planners.

▶ Conclusion

The spread of diseases globally poses a risk to the nation's health and security. The U.S. government has developed strategies to help protect the health of the nation during emergencies. In particular, the NHSS is designed to guide the nation's efforts to minimize the risks associated with a wide range of potential large-scale incidents that put the health and well-being of the nation's people at risk. State and local emergency planners must be diligent in their efforts to effectively plan and prepare to protect the nation from pandemic influenza threats. As has been seen over the last century, pandemics take many years to occur, but they do occur. When that happens, most of the population will have little to no immunity against the pandemic strain. Thus, public health officials need to constantly plan for mitigation of this deadly threat.

Discussion Questions

1. Why is global connectedness a threat to health security?
2. What is pandemic influenza? Why should the occurrence of pandemics be of such great concern to emergency planners?
3. Name the three pandemics that occurred in the 20th century. Which of these was the deadliest and why?
4. What is antigenic drift? Antigenic shift? During which of these events does a major pandemic occur?
5. What are some common societal disruptions that result from an influenza pandemic?

References

1. World Health Organization. Avian and other zoonotic influenza. Available at http://www.who.int/mediacentre/factsheets/avian_influenza/en/. Accessed July 21, 2017.
2. Katz R. *Essentials of Public Health Preparedness*. Burlington, MA: Jones & Bartlett Learning; 2013.
3. National Healthcare Security Strategy of the United States, p. 3. December 2009. Available at http://www.phe.gov/Preparedness/planning/authority/nhss/strategy/Documents/nhss-final.pdf. Accessed April 4, 2017.
4. Heymann DL, Rodier G. Global surveillance, national surveillance, and SARS. *Emerg Infect Diseases*. 2004;10(2):173–175. doi:10.3201/eid1002.031038.
5. Landesman LY. *Public Health Management of Disasters*. 2nd ed. Washington, DC: American Public Health Association.
6. Taubenberger JK, Morens DM. The pathology of influenza virus infections. *Annu Rev Pathol*. 2008;3:499–522. doi:10.1146/annurev.pathmechdis.3.121806.154316.
7. Contra Costa Health Services. Public Health Division. Pandemic influenza presentation. 2006. Available at www.cchealth.org/pandemic-flu/school-action-kit/pandemic_flu_preso.ppt. Accessed April 4, 2017.
8. U.S. Centers for Disease Control and Prevention. How the flu virus can change: "Drift" and "Shift". Available at https://www.cdc.gov/flu/about/viruses/change.htm. Accessed April 4, 2017.
9. Glezen WP. Emerging infections: pandemic influenza. *Epidemiol Rev*. 1996;18:65. Available at https://pdfs.semanticscholar.org/d59b/9e698f7830bdcd1aa577d453e9c02bc24da3.pdf. Accessed April 4, 2017.

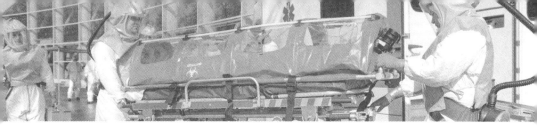

CHAPTER 6

Epidemiology and Surveillance in Preparedness and Response

LEARNING OBJECTIVES

Epidemiology and surveillance are hallmarks of public health emergency response. Particularly with respect to large-scale outbreaks, whether foodborne or infectious disease outbreaks, epidemiological and surveillance tools assist public health responders in determining the cause of the outbreak, commonalities among those affected, and interventions for mitigation. The information obtained through epidemiological investigations drives public health response actions. By the end of this chapter, readers should be able to:

- Define epidemiology and surveillance
- Describe the importance of epidemiological investigations in response to emergencies and disasters
- Distinguish the difference between multiple types of surveillance activities
- Describe disease surveillance systems, tools, networks, and processes
- Understand the use of surveillance information in decision-making
- Articulate the importance of ethical principles in decision-making during preparedness for and response to emergencies

▶ What Is Epidemiology?

Epidemiology is defined as the study of diseases and injuries in human populations, disease patterns, and the frequency of occurrence. It is the scientific method of problem solving used by epidemiologists, lab scientists, statisticians, and physicians to understand the origins and causes of disease in a community. Epidemiology is considered to be the basic science of public health.[1]

Epidemiologists carry out several critical functions during outbreaks of infectious disease, including:

- Conducting epidemiological investigations
- Determining risk of exposure for various populations
- Identifying populations in need of prophylaxis
- Providing recommendations to the healthcare community and public
- Determining criteria to be used for identification of cases and controls
- Monitoring morbidity and mortality associated with the emergency

▶ Outbreak Investigations

Outbreaks occur when an increased number of cases of disease have been identified within a time frame that is unusual or unexpected at any given time. The purpose of the outbreak investigation is to quickly identify the cause of the outbreak and suggest interventions to minimize additional disease occurrence.[1] In the wake of an outbreak, public health professionals will begin the process of investigation to determine the cause and, in many cases, to identify and define the type of outbreak. An investigation can involve interviewing all affected people to identify commonalities in their histories. For example, have all people who report similar symptoms consumed the same food in the recent past? Have they all recently traveled to a specific location? Have they all interacted with a specific kind of animal recently?

Some outbreaks can be traced to their origins quickly in an epidemiological investigation. For example, in January 2015, the California Department of Public Health received a report of a suspected measles case. The patient's only notable travel history was a recent trip to a Disney theme park. That same day, four more cases appeared, and epidemiologists quickly discovered that all of the patients had recently visited the same park. The outbreak ultimately sickened 125 patients and is believed to have been caused by international visitors from countries where measles is endemic and spread by persons both vaccinated and unvaccinated. This outbreak represents an incident that was quickly traced to its origin.[2]

Cases of Middle East respiratory syndrome (MERS) and severe acute respiratory syndrome (SARS), both coronaviruses, are examples of other infectious diseases that have spread globally due to international travel. The United States reported its first case of MERS in May 2014 after a traveler from Saudi Arabia traveled to the United States while symptomatic. In 2003, more than 8000 people around the world became ill with SARS, including eight in the United States. Of the total infected, 774 died. Both of these outbreaks were controlled in the United States with the help of careful surveillance, which we discuss in more detail later in this chapter.

Ebola and other viral hemorrhagic fevers are diseases that can be highly infectious and require a swift and thorough investigation. These diseases affect multiple organ systems in the body and can frequently be life threatening without early intervention. In March 2014, Ebola was reported in a region of southeastern

Guinea and spread rapidly throughout West Africa, particularly in Guinea, Liberia, and Sierra Leone. The outbreak lasted for more than a year, killed more than 11,000 patients, and sickened hundreds of thousands more. This outbreak also represented a significant global health threat that spread beyond West Africa. After a Liberian man traveled to Texas without disclosing his contact with an infected patient in Liberia, he began exhibiting symptoms and was admitted to a Dallas hospital. Eventually, he became the first person in the United States to be diagnosed with Ebola and subsequently infected two nurses, who became the first cases of Ebola transmission in the United States.[3]

▶ The Role of Social Epidemiology

Social epidemiology is an important approach to investigating infectious diseases. This branch of epidemiology focuses on how social, cultural, and economic—rather than biological—circumstances affect the state of health of specific populations. A robust understanding of social epidemiology should inform all preparedness planning by public health practitioners.

We know that social, political, behavioral, and environmental factors shape the emergence and reemergence of infectious diseases,[2] such as Ebola, AIDS, and tuberculosis.[4] When social factors are taken into consideration during development of preparedness plans, public health systems are better able to track the origins of outbreaks, contain disease from spreading, and anticipate both the effects of an outbreak on a specific population, as well as circumstances that may compound response efforts.

For example, when Hurricane Katrina hit the Gulf Coast in August 2005, one of the worst affected areas was the low-lying Lower Ninth Ward of New Orleans. The Lower Ninth Ward was vulnerable to the flooding that ultimately inundated its boundaries, not only due to its geography but also because of its high level of poverty. This ward was one of the city's poorest neighborhoods and predominantly African American. Its population was predisposed to certain chronic health conditions, such as diabetes and high blood pressure.[5,6] Due to underlying health conditions, among other social factors, residents in this area were also less likely to evacuate before the flooding began. These circumstances combined with the natural disaster to create favorable conditions for the spread of certain infectious diseases, such as methicillin-resistant *Staphylococcus aureus* and infection by waterborne pathogens such as *Vibrio vulnificus*, related to the bacteria that causes cholera. Approximately, 1000 cases of diarrhea and vomiting were reported among evacuees in Mississippi and Texas.[7] The occurrence of these symptoms had to be managed, while responders were also involved in response to the hurricane. In incidents such as these, social epidemiology can predict populations that will be more susceptible to infectious disease and work to prevent their occurrence or mitigate their spread.

▶ The Role of Surveillance

Along with epidemiology, surveillance is understood to be the second scientific pillar of public health. Surveillance refers to the collection, analysis, interpretation, and dissemination of data on disease occurrence. Surveillance can be passive, in which health systems are collecting and reporting data to a public health department, or active, in which epidemiologists are proactively seeking and gathering data for an investigation. Global disease threats require diligent surveillance activity to protect countries from large-scale emerging and reemerging infectious disease outbreaks.

Several outbreaks over the last decade of the *20th* century have demonstrated the consequences that delayed national recognition and response to outbreaks can have: "illness and death of national populations including health workers, potential spread to other countries, and significant disruptions of travel and trade."[8] Inadequate surveillance and response capability in one area of the world can endanger national populations and the public health security of the entire world.

The data collected through surveillance may come from a variety of sources, including community medical providers, hospital emergency departments and healthcare systems (syndromic surveillance), sentinel surveillance systems, zoonotic surveillance, and other data reporting systems. Surveillance almost always involves cooperation among multiple entities, so the partnerships and necessary systems for reporting must be in place prior to an emergency to ensure seamless availability of information.

▶ Types of Surveillance

Syndromic surveillance is the use of data from healthcare providers, in real time, to investigate and analyze potential outbreaks. A passive form of surveillance, it was originally developed as a means to detect a large-scale release of a biological agent, but today the goals of syndromic surveillance extend far beyond preparing for a terrorist event.[9] The overarching goal is to use real-time data to identify illness clusters before diagnoses are even confirmed or reported to public health agencies. This type of surveillance focuses on data about symptoms in the earliest stages of an illness. Syndromic surveillance may also collect surrogate data such as reported absences from school or work, veterinary data such as unexpected avian deaths, or even social media posts about illness.[10]

Sentinel surveillance is an active form of surveillance and involves the collection of data from a carefully selected sampling of reporting sites. Selected healthcare providers agree to report cases of specific illnesses to a central health department on a regular basis. Sites must be willing to serve as sentinels; be located near or in a relatively large population; have the staff and expertise to diagnose, treat, and report cases of the disease they are monitoring; and have a high-quality diagnostics laboratory. Data collected at sentinel sites can be used by epidemiologists and public health departments to identify trends and outbreaks in a more cost-effective way than traditional Types of Surveillance.

Zoonotic surveillance systems collect data on animals infected with diseases that can be transmitted to humans. One such example is ArboNET, a passive national surveillance system managed by the Centers for Disease Control and Prevention (CDC) and state health departments. ArboNET collects data on veterinary disease cases, dead birds, mosquitos, sentinel animals, and presumptive viremic blood donors (PVDs).[11] ArboNET is critical in the surveillance of diseases such as Zika virus, West Nile virus, Chikungunya fever, Dengue fever, Yellow fever, and Japanese encephalitis.

▶ Role of Laboratories

Public health laboratories are another critical component for identifying threats to the public's health. They are responsible for assuring laboratory services in support of public health, including preparedness and response.[12] During the conduct of epidemiological disease investigations, specimens are often collected for the purpose of laboratory testing. This aids in the identification process for determining the cause of an outbreak. For preparedness and response purposes, local and state public health laboratories must maintain the ability to "conduct rapid and conventional detection, characterization, confirmatory testing, data reporting, investigative support and laboratory networking to address actual or potential exposure to all hazards."[13]

▶ Laboratory Response Network

In 1999, the Laboratory Response Network (LRN) was formed. The LRN is a national system of more than 150 sentinel laboratories that provide rapid detection of, and response to, threats related to chemical, biological, and radiological threats as well as natural disasters. Founded by the Association of Public Health Laboratories, CDC, and the Federal Bureau of Investigation to advance national readiness for bioterrorist threats. The LRN's members include local, state, and federal public health laboratories, food testing laboratories, veterinary diagnostic laboratories, and environmental testing laboratories.[14,15]

The LRN establishes standard protocols to identify dangerous pathogens, provides guidelines for the safe handling of suspected threat agents, identifies threats using complex molecular identification, and provides expert advice. Since its inception, the LRN has responded to multiple threats, including avian influenza, the anthrax attacks of 2001, and SARS.

▶ National Strategy for Biosurveillance

In 2012, the Department of Homeland Security, under President Barack Obama, released the National Strategy for Biosurveillance. The directive called for the creation of a networked system of federal, state, local, and tribal governments; private-sector businesses; nongovernmental organizations, and international partners that can cooperate to collect and report timely data on infectious, toxic, and metabolic threats to human and animal health. Including a number of guiding principles, the strategy defined an approach to the nation's biosurveillance efforts aimed at addressing both short-term and long-term information needs for decision makers at all levels of government. The Guiding Principles of the strategy included:

- ■ "Leverage Existing Capabilities
- ■ Embrace an All-of-Nation Approach [to biosurveillance]
- ■ Add Value for All Participants
- ■ Maintain a Global Health Perspective"[16]

▶ Ethical Considerations in Decision-Making

Disasters and public health emergencies can be overwhelming to health systems. By definition, they can affect large portions of the public rather than just an individual, which means the normal operation of public health infrastructure will not be adequate. Needs will often surpass available resources. As a result, practitioners may be faced with countless ethical dilemmas.

These dilemmas can relate to prioritization of patient treatment, rationing of supplies, risks to the lives of first responders, evacuation decisions, and how to handle uncooperative members of the public. For example, if you have only one respirator and two sick patients, who gets the respirator? When is it ethical to move from a rescue effort to a recovery effort? Who should be evacuated from a danger zone first? How should you balance a person's right to refuse treatment with the public interest? When is it acceptable to declare and enforce a curfew that infringes on the public's right to move freely? These types of decisions are extremely consequential, can be a matter of life and death, and therefore should not be decided in the midst of a crisis.

Because normal levels of healthcare services cannot be assured in disasters, public health systems must do what they can to gain the trust of the public by responding fairly and equitably, particularly for the most vulnerable populations.[17] This requires conscientious and systematic preparation to ensure that:

- The response offers the best care possible given the resources on hand
- Decisions are fair and transparent
- Policies and protocols within and across states are consistent
- Citizens and stakeholders are included and heard[18]

In 2009, the Institute of Medicine (IOM) convened a panel of experts to develop Crisis Standards of Care (CSC), an extensive national framework that establishes standards of care to be applied in disaster situations of all types. The change in care standards become justified when a disaster or emergency renders a healthcare system incapable of meeting normal standards. After a formal government declaration, crisis operations remain in effect for a certain period of time.

This framework contains volumes targeted at multiple functional areas, including state and local governments, emergency medical services, hospitals, alternate care systems, and public engagement. The guidelines for use by state and local public health officials and institutions include six key recommendations and provide a template for addressing legal issues, ethical considerations, palliative care, and mental health treatment when normal healthcare operations and the normal level of care are impossible to maintain.

The six recommendations include the development of CSC protocols that encompass the following:

- "A strong ethical grounding, ensuring fairness, transparency, consistency, proportionality, and accountability
- Community and provider engagement, education, and communication
- The necessary legal assurances that CSC can be ethically implemented without legal repercussion
- Clear indicators, triggers for declaring crisis operations, and lines of responsibility
- Evidence-based clinical processes and operations"[18]

Above all in preparedness planning, it is incumbent on public health practitioners to ensure that vulnerable populations are treated fairly and ethically. These populations may be considered vulnerable because of their age, underlying health conditions, socioeconomic status, disability, or even limited English proficiency, and any CSC plan must address these populations specifically.

▶ Conclusion

Epidemiology and surveillance are the hallmarks of public health emergency response. The goals of epidemiology and surveillance are to identify the source or cause of disease, determine if additional risks of infection still exist, disseminate information about the source of the infection, provide treatment recommendations to minimize morbidity and mortality, and monitor cases to ensure the treatment modalities are being effective against the infection. Epidemiologists also collect specimens for the purpose of laboratory testing. Public health laboratories aid in the identification process for determining the cause of an outbreak. For threats of public health significance, such as pandemic influenza, bioterrorism agents, and highly pathogenic infectious diseases, it is critical that public health laboratories are networked and integrated to ensure rapid identification of and response to these threats.

Large-scale public health threats have the potential to overwhelm healthcare facilities and systems. At times, resources may begin to dwindle and the ability to provide care to all those in need could become increasingly difficult, perhaps due to facility damage or less than ideal conditions. These situations require advance planning that is conducted based on ethical guidelines to ensure standards of care that can be applied in disaster situations. When planning for dire situations is completed in advance, decision makers can make more informed decisions that are grounded in ethical principles.

Discussion Questions

1. What is epidemiology?
2. Why are epidemiology and surveillance critical to emergency preparedness and response?
3. Describe the potential effect of SARS in the United States without robust surveillance capability.
4. What are some of the advantages of an integrated laboratory network, such as the LRN?

References

1. Dworkin M. *Cases in Field Epidemiology: A Global Perspective.* 1st ed. Burlington, MA: Jones & Bartlett Learning; 2011.
2. U.S. Centers for Disease Control. Measles outbreak – California, December 2014–February 2015. *MMWR.* February 20, 2015;64(06):153–154.
3. U.S. Centers for Disease Control. Ebola virus disease cluster in the United States – Dallas County, Texas, 2014. *MMWR.* November 14, 2014;63(Early release):1–3.
4. Heymann DL. Social, behavioural and environmental factors and their impact on infectious disease outbreaks. *J Public Health Policy.* 2005 Apr;26(1):133–139.

5. Farmer P. Social inequalities and emerging infectious diseases. *Emerg Infect Dis.* 1996;2(4):259–269.
6. New Orleans after the Storm: lessons from the past, a plan for the future. The Brookings Institution Metropolitan Policy Program, 2015. Available at https://www.brookings.edu /wp-content/uploads/2016/06/20051012_NewOrleans.pdf.
7. Infectious disease and dermatologic conditions in evacuees and rescue workers after Hurricane Katrina—multiple states, August–September, 2005. *MMWR.* September 30, 2005;54(38):961–964. Available at https://www.cdc.gov/mmwr/preview/mmwrhtml /mm5438a6.htm.
8. Heyman DL, Rodier G. Global surveillance, national surveillance, and SARS. *Emerg Infect Diseases.* 2004;10(2):173–175. Available at http://wwwnc.cdc.gov/eid/article/10/2/03-1038.htm.
9. Overview of syndromic surveillance: what is syndromic surveillance? *MMWR.* September 24, 2004;53(Suppl):5–11. Available at https://www.cdc.gov/mmwr/preview/mmwrhtml /su5301a3.htm.
10. Coberly JS, Fink CR, Elbert E, et al. Tweeting fever: are tweet extracts a valid surrogate data source for dengue fever? *Online J Public Health Inf.* 2013;5(1):e64. Available at https://www .ncbi.nlm.nih.gov/pmc/articles/PMC3692911/.
11. U.S. Centers for Disease Control and Prevention. ArboNET. Available at https://www.cdc .gov/westnile/resourcepages/survresources.html.
12. The core functions of public health laboratories, association of public health laboratories, 2014. Available at https://www.aphl.org/aboutaphl/publications/documents /aphlcorefunctionsandcapabilities_2014.pdf.
13. Public health preparedness capabilities: national standards for state and local planning, U.S. Centers for Disease Control and Prevention, March 2011. Available at https://www.cdc.gov /phpr/readiness/00_docs/DSLR_capabilities_July.pdf.
14. FAQs about the Laboratory Response Network (LRN). Available at https://emergency.cdc .gov/lrn/faq.asp.
15. Public health laboratories: leveraging partnerships to strengthen preparedness and response. Association of Public Health Laboratories. May 2013. Available at https://www .aphl.org/aboutAPHL/publications/Documents/PHPR_2013May_All-Hazards-Laboratory -Preparedness-Report_Leveraging-Partnerships-to-Strengthen-Preparedness-and-Response.pdf.
16. National Strategy for Biosurveillance. 2012. Available at https://obamawhitehouse.archives .gov/sites/default/files/National_Strategy_for_Biosurveillance_July_2012.pdf.
17. Lawrence O. Gostin, Madison Powers. What does social justice require for the public's health: public health ethics and policy imperatives. *Health Aff.* Jul/Aug 2006;25(4):1053 (Health Module).
18. Institute of Medicine (IOM). 2009. *Guidance for Establishing Crisis Standards of Care for Use in Disaster Situations: A Letter Report.* Washington, DC: The National Academies Press. Available at http://www.iom.edu/Reports/2009/DisasterCareStandards.aspx.

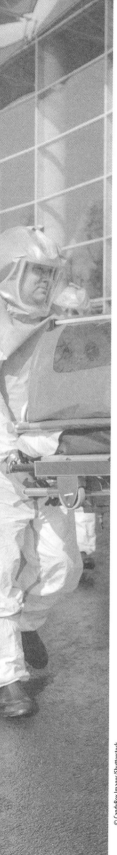

PART III

The Preparedness Cycle

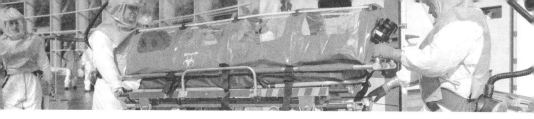

CHAPTER 7

Hazard Assessment and Planning

LEARNING OBJECTIVES

Preparedness can sometimes be misconstrued as a destination or outcome. In fact, due to the constantly changing nature of factors that affect preparedness—social, political, economic, and environmental—a community's level of preparedness can change day to day. For this reason, it is critical that public health practitioners approach preparedness with a flexible mindset. Practitioners must also understand the specific hazards and threats for which they need to be prepared, as well as have processes in place to properly plan for and develop readiness to mitigate these hazards and threats. Above all, it is important to remember that preparedness is a journey, never a destination. By the end of this chapter, readers should be able to:

- Describe each component of the preparedness cycle
- Understand the importance of assessing risks as a critical component of preparedness
- Describe the purpose of a hazard vulnerability assessment (HVA) and the basic processes for completing an HVA
- Articulate the various types of emergency operations plans (EOPs)
- Identify several types of vulnerable or at-risk populations and specific considerations that should made for these groups during the planning process
- Define the whole community approach to preparedness, and apply this approach to an emergency situation

▶ Planning and Preparing for Disasters

The Department of Homeland Security's Federal Emergency Management Agency (FEMA) defines preparedness as a "continuous cycle of planning, organizing, training, exercising, evaluating and taking corrective action in an effort to ensure effective coordination during incident response."[1] As the cycle is completed, organizations take findings from the evaluation phase and circle back into the planning phase, ever strengthening their ability to be as prepared as possible.

The preparedness cycle, as it is called, is frequently graphically demonstrated to outline how the process is used by the whole community to guide preparedness activities (see **FIGURE 7-1**).[2] As jurisdictions strive to more closely integrate the principles

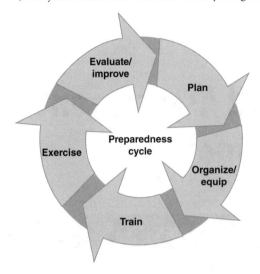

FIGURE 7-1 The preparedness cycle

Data from Federal Emergency Management Agency. Preparedness Cycle. Available at: www.fema.gov/media-library/assets/images/114295#. Accessed August 29, 2017.

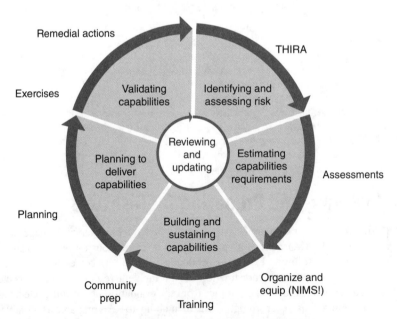

FIGURE 7-2 The preparedness cycle: National Preparedness System version

Data from the "National Incident Management System Update"; M. Bernard. FEMA Region X. April 2012.

of the National Incident Management System (NIMS) into their preparedness activities, a more detailed depiction of the preparedness cycle includes assessment as the first step in the cycle, and also considers capability development and community inclusion as critical elements in the cycle (see **FIGURE 7-2**).

In this chapter, we examine the ways in which communities must assess preparedness and begin planning for disaster. In other chapters, we explore the remainder of the preparedness cycle in detail.

▶ Assessing Risk

The first step in the preparedness cycle is conducting an assessment to understand the particular risks a community faces. Assessments are designed to identify vulnerabilities to possible disaster scenarios, determine a jurisdiction's ability to respond to and mitigate the risks of a disaster, and help the jurisdiction prioritize which elements of preparation need improvement. Only after an assessment can public health practitioners develop plans to address the hazards or threats identified by the assessment.

Hazard Vulnerability Assessments

An HVA is a systematic approach to identifying all hazards that may affect a jurisdiction, community, or organization, assessing the probability of occurrence associated with each hazard, and analyzing findings using mathematical calculations to create a prioritized comparison of hazard vulnerabilities.[3]

HVAs define all possible hazards that could affect a community. HVAs also provide the basis for mitigation strategies that are taken to ensure effective recovery from emergencies and disasters. As described by FEMA, "the four basic components of a hazard assessment are: (1) hazard identification, (2) profiling of hazard events, (3) inventory of assets, and (4) estimation of potential human and economic losses based on the exposure and vulnerability of people, buildings, and infrastructure."[4] Naturally, hazard assessments should focus on protection of human assets from emergencies and disasters; however, other assets are also important. Physical assets such as buildings, utilities, information systems, and supply chain systems should also be carefully considered,[5] as well as the impacts to these assets if subjected to damage.

Once potential hazards have been identified, an HVA then assigns a likelihood of each event occurring, from low to moderate to high. The likelihood of occurrence may be calculated using hard data, such as statistics, and historical data regarding how often that event has occurred in the past. Probability may also be intuitive or based on subjective information. For example, it is possible that a hospital located far from urban areas and far from nuclear power plants could nonetheless be affected by a nuclear detonation. And although there may be no available statistical data to assign probability of radiation exposure in such a location, it is reasonable to subjectively assume that the probability is quite low.

An HVA next calculates the severity of impact—from low to moderate to high—that a given event would have on humans, property, and the ability to continue operations. It may also take into account factors such as financial impact, legal issues, and impact on community trust.

These data are then analyzed to determine a level of preparedness related to each potential hazard. The resulting scores help a community or organization prioritize its efforts to minimize vulnerabilities to the identified hazards. For example, a facility may be well prepared to respond to seasonal influenza but find that it is ill prepared to respond to a large-scale water contamination event. Resources may then be directed toward scaling up preparedness around water contamination events.

The Risk Assessment Process Diagram shown in **FIGURE 7-3** illustrates the close relationship and interdependencies between hazards, assets, and the impact on those assets.

In addition to communities and jurisdictions, organizations such as hospitals can use HVAs to assess risks within their organizations. Since the events of September 11, 2001, the Joint Commission (formerly the Joint Commission on Accreditation of Healthcare Organizations) has required accredited hospitals to complete HVAs, but other types of organizations frequently develop HVAs as the first step in preparedness planning. Organizations that would benefit from an HVA include health departments, public transportation systems, and any type of healthcare facility that may need to respond in the event of a disaster.

The use of HVAs within organizations can ensure identification of broad threats that have a high potential of occurrence, and can also identify additional threats due to social, environmental, or other factors. For example, an HVA for a hospital system in Florida would include many threats with the potential to affect any community, such as foodborne outbreaks, infectious disease outbreaks, power outages, hostage situations, and terrorist attacks. That same HVA, however, could also identify other hazards such as hurricanes, flooding, Zika, and extreme heat, as direct possibilities based on Florida's unique characteristics and geography.

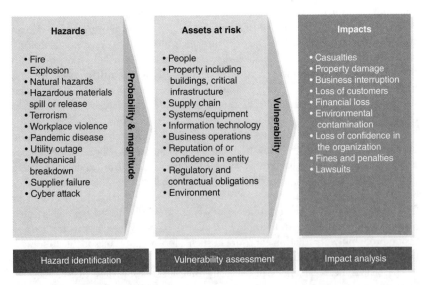

FIGURE 7-3 Risk Assessment Process Diagram

Data from Department of Homeland Security. Risk Assessment. Available at: www.ready.gov/risk-assessment. Accessed August 28, 2017.

Threat and Hazard Identification and Risk Assessment (THIRA)

While the HVA is an ideal tool for assessing vulnerabilities of constrained systems, its results are specific to a single facility or organization and cannot be accurately extrapolated or applied to a larger community involving multiple response partners. The THIRA is a model that is better suited to determining the preparedness of larger communities such as cities, counties, and states and the large number of responder organizations associated with them.

The THIRA process should take a whole community approach, seeking input from government agencies, academia, nonprofits, businesses, faith-based organizations, and key individuals. The process follows five specific steps:

1. **"Identify the threats and hazards of concern.** Based on past experiences, future predictions and expert assessment, identify all the threats and hazards that could potentially impact the community.
2. **Give the threats and hazards context.** Using that list, add context that describes *how* those threats and hazards could affect the community.
3. **Examine the capabilities using the threats and hazards.** Using the context, define all potential impacts to the community in terms of core capabilities outlined in the National Preparedness Goal[6] (see **TABLE 7-1**).
4. **Establish capability targets.** For each potential impact, and based on desired outcomes, set capability targets.
5. **Apply the results.** Plan for the ability to meet capability targets with either community assets or mutual aid, identify mitigation opportunities and drive preparedness activities."[7]

The objective of the THIRA process is similar to the HVA process: to develop a strategy to direct resources according to the greatest need for reducing risk. If resources are inadequate, a jurisdiction may be able to seek additional funding, such as applying for federal grants, to achieve capability targets. By taking a whole-community approach,[7] the THIRA not only reflects a comprehensive understanding of the community but it also can leverage available expertise. The THIRA process must be continuous so that it can adapt to changes in the community or changes in the likelihood of specific threats.

▶ National Preparedness Goal Core Capabilities

In 2015, President Barack Obama signed Presidential Policy Directive-8: National Preparedness, a document that describes an approach to preparing for threats and hazards. This directive outlines 32 core capabilities grouped into five categories.

TABLE 7-1 Core Capabilities of the National Preparedness Goal

Capability	Prevention	Protection	Mitigation	Response	Recovery
Planning	X	X	X	X	X
Public information and warning	X	X	X	X	X
Operational coordination	X	X	X	X	X
Forensics and attribution	X				
Intelligence and information sharing	X	X			
Interdiction and disruption	X	X			
Screening, search, and detection	X	X			
Access control and identity verification		X			
Cybersecurity		X			
Physical protective measures		X			
Risk management for protection programs and activities		X			
Supply chain integrity and security		X			
Community resilience			X		
Long-term vulnerability reduction			X		
Risk and disaster resilience assessment			X		
Threats and hazard identification			X		

TABLE 7-1 Core Capabilities of the National Preparedness Goal

Capability	Prevention	Protection	Mitigation	Response	Recovery
Critical transportation				X	
Environmental response/health and safety				X	
Fatality management services				X	
Fire management and suppression				X	
Infrastructure systems				X	X
Logistics and supply chain management				X	
Mass care services				X	
Mass search and rescue operations				X	
On-scene security, protection, and law enforcement				X	
Operational communications				X	
Public health, healthcare, and emergency medical services				X	
Situational assessment				X	
Economic recovery					X
Health and social services					X
Housing					X
Natural and cultural resources					X

Let's take a more in-depth look at the five steps of the THIRA process.

Step 1: Identify Threats and Hazards of Concern

Communities should include all threats that may affect them, whether natural, technological, or caused by humans. Existing threat assessments may be useful in this step, as they will outline threats that local organizations have already identified. Other potential data sources include U.S Geological Survey, Census Bureau, Environmental Protection Agency, National Counterterrorism Center, National Weather Services, local fire and police departments, colleges and universities, and tribal governments.

It is important to consider threats in neighboring communities that may also affect a jurisdiction. For example, a chemical spill in one community may affect multiple communities downwind. Likewise, an inland community may not be directly hit by hurricanes but might become inundated with coastal residents fleeing an affected area.

Step 2: Give the Threats and Hazards Context

This step is intended to provide a more complete picture of the context in which each potential threat may become a reality. In certain cases, a jurisdiction may need to describe multiple contexts. All possibilities of reasonable likelihood must be considered and addressed individually, because they will require different responses and may indicate different levels of preparedness. Here are two examples:

Example 1: Coastal city prone to hurricanes

Threat Group: Natural

Threat Type: Hurricane

Description 1: A Category 3 hurricane makes landfall in the afternoon in a heavily touristed area during peak tourist season.

Description 2: A Category 4 hurricane makes landfall overnight in a low-lying area populated largely by poor residents.

Example 2: Mid-sized city

Threat Group: Technological

Threat Type: Train derailment with hazardous material release

Description 1: A train derails and releases hazardous material in a heavily populated residential area on a summer weekend.

Description 2: A train derails and releases hazardous material in a rural area near the city's borders and threatens to contaminate groundwater sources.

Context can change over time based on changes in demographics, climate, political factors, and construction and development. When any of those factors changes, jurisdictions must revisit this step of the THIRA.

Step 3: Examine the Core Capabilities Using the Threats and Hazards

This step entails determining how each threat could impact the community, and pairing potential impacts with desired outcomes. The objective is to begin

TABLE 7-2 Core Capabilities and Desired Outcomes for a Hurricane	
Core Capability	**Desired Outcome**
Long-term vulnerability reduction	Complete a necessary upgrade and modernization of levee systems in low-lying areas over next 5 years
Public information and warning	Expand hurricane warning siren coverage of coastal areas within 1 year
	Increase availability of public-facing hurricane preparedness documents translated into Spanish, French, German, Arabic, and Mandarin; distribute to tourist destinations and residential areas as needed within 6 months
Fatality management services	During the first 72 hours post-landfall, conduct operations to recover fatalities

understanding what must be done to make achievement of those outcomes possible. Well-defined outcomes should include specific actions to be taken, as well as projected timelines for completion of the activity.

Each desired outcome must be viewed through the lens of the capabilities listed in the National Preparedness Goals. For example, **TABLE 7-2** presents possible desired outcomes from a hurricane.

This information will help jurisdictions to determine estimated impacts. An example of various scenarios and their impacts, as viewed through the lens of the core capabilities, is shown in **TABLE 7-3**.[7]

Step 4: Set Capability Targets

After determining desired outcomes and estimating impacts, this step involves combining the two to create capability targets. For example, if the greatest impact of an improvised explosive device (IED) attack is estimated to be 52 fatalities, and the desired outcome is to recover all fatalities within 72 hours after an attack, the capability target will be as follows: *During the first 72 hours of an attack, search for and recover 52 fatalities.*

Step 5: Apply the Results

Finally, the result of the THIRA must be applied to mitigation and preparedness efforts. This step may include:

- Determining the resources required to achieve capability targets
- Filling gaps in capabilities through partnership with other local agencies, regional offices of national agencies, faith-based organizations, nongovernmental organizations, and so on
- Seeking available grants or other funding sources
- Briefing community leaders, government officials, and the public

TABLE 7-3 Estimated Impacts for Core Capabilities

	Prevention	Protection	Mitigation	Response		Recovery	
	Screening, Search, and Detection	Access Control and Identity Verification	Long-term Vulnerability Reduction	Fatality Management Services	Public Health and Medical Services	Infrastructure Systems	Economic Recovery
IED Attack: A lone actor deploys an improvised explosive device (IED) in an indoor concourse of a stadium during a sporting event	**67,500 spectators 2,500 vendors and employees**	**2,500 vendor and employees**	Reinforce 500 concrete support columns in stadium concourse	52 fatalities	350 casualties	N/A	$14 million of direct economic loss (ticket sales, hotel stays, parking, food, and souvenirs)
Accidental Chemical Material Release: A nighttime accident in the rail yard results in the release of a toxic inhalation hazard (TIH) in a densely populated residential area	N/A	350 rail yard employees and first responders	**Reroute 100% of rail carrying TIH around densely populated areas**	4 fatalities	75 casualties	Damage and contamination to 3 lines at the rail yard	$11 million or direct economic loss (loss of the chemical, physical damage to train, damage to rail yard)
Earthquake: A magnitude 7.2 earthquake centered near an urban area occurs during mid-afternoon in March	N/A	N/A	Undertake seismic retrofit measures at all public stadiums	**375 fatalities**	**8,400 casualties**	**350,000 customers without power**	**$8.4 billion of direct economic loss**

Community Risk Assessment

After the creation of an HVA, it is necessary to assess the risk a community faces under each identified threat and create a plan for each hazard. The four steps of community risk assessment include the following:

1. Identify hazardous sites and transportation routes
2. Identify potential incident scenarios
3. Identify vulnerable populations
4. Estimate the health impacts of potential incidents

For example, a community in Tornado Alley in the Midwestern United States will need to develop a tornado response plan. Hazardous sites might include water filtration plants, hospitals, and nuclear power plants. Hazardous transportation routes could include main thoroughfares lined by trees or power poles that could be knocked down during a tornado, making routes impassable. Potential incident scenarios might include a tornado traveling through a residential area or through a busy downtown business district. Vulnerable populations might include the elderly, the physically disabled, hospital patients, inmates held in jails or prisons, school-children, or those with limited English proficiency. Health impacts could include a high number of casualties, and power outages affecting healthcare facilities and impassable roads that block emergency responders. It is necessary to create response plans for every threat identified in an HVA.

Rapid Needs Assessments

Rapid needs assessments (RNAs, also called rapid health assessments) are most often conducted in conjunction with emergency response efforts to determine the specific health impact of a disaster on a specific community, *after the disaster has occurred*. RNA teams collect, analyze, and disseminate data that are timely and accurate to assist public health practitioners and first responders in determining immediate health needs and response actions.

In the immediate aftermath of the deadly Indian Ocean tsunami of December 2004, government and humanitarian organizations on the ground collected data about mortality, casualties, the viability of the local healthcare system, the state of sewage systems, and the adequacy of medical supplies and morgue facilities. The objective of collecting this information post disaster is to provide these data to those involved in emergency response so they can respond more effectively to conditions on the ground as they are unfolding.

▶ Planning

The next stage of the preparedness cycle intentionally builds on the discoveries of the assessment stage. Organizations create emergency operations plans (EOPs) for each hazard identified during the assessment stage that incorporate its needs, vulnerabilities, and existing capabilities. Planning is an extensive process that must be revisited after organizations complete further stages of the preparedness cycle.

Emergency Operations Plans

EOPs are detailed documents that describe the actions an organization or emergency response system will undertake to mitigate the effects of, and recover from, specific disasters. The goal of an EOP is to:

- "Assign responsibility to people and organizations for carrying out actions related to the emergency
- Identify roles and responsibilities of staff responding under the plan
- Provide lines of authority for execution of the plan
- Identify available resources to mitigate the emergency"[8(pp2-6)]

EOPs may borrow the same basic plan for all disasters, but their annexes will include different details for each specific threat. For example, the complete EOP for a foodborne disease outbreak would be dramatically different from a complete EOP for an active shooter situation.

In 2010, the FEMA released Comprehensive Preparedness Guide (CPG) 101 to provide guidance for developing EOPs.[8] CPG 101 outlines the steps involved in EOP development, which include:

- Form a collaborative planning team
- Understand the situation
- Determine goals and objectives for the plan
- Develop the plan and solutions to address the problem
- Submit the plan for review and approval
- Implement and maintain the plan

Several formats can be used when developing EOPs. A functional or traditional format includes three basic sections: basic plan, functional annexes, and hazard-specific annexes. An Emergency Support Function (ESF) format includes a basic plan as well as individual ESF annexes. Finally, an agency-focused format addresses the tasks of an agency or department.[8] **FIGURES 7-4** through **7-6** illustrate the components of each of these formats.

Continuity of Operations Plans

Continuity of Operations Plans (COOPs) define an organization's ability to perform its essential functions continuously during an emergency event or resume them quickly after an emergency.[9] The plan describes how an organization will meet its continuity responsibilities, how work will continue to be done, which positions and personnel will be needed, which nonessential functions can be discontinued until the crisis is over, how vital records will be preserved, what alternative worksites can be used, and more.[10]

A continuity plan must address four phases:

1. **Readiness and preparation:** Planning, coordinating, testing, and improving emergency plans
2. **Activation and relocation:** 0–12 hours post-emergency
3. **Continuity of operations:** As soon as routine operations can be resumed, somewhere between 12 hours and 30 days
4. **Reconstitution:** Recovery, mitigation, and termination

TRADITIONAL FUNCTIONAL EOP FORMAT

❶ Basic Plan

- a) Introductory Material
  - (i) Promulgation Document/ Signatures
  - (ii) Approval and Implementation
  - (iii) Record of Changes
  - (iv) Record of Distribution
  - (v) Table of Contents
- b) Purpose, Scope, Situation Overview, and Assumptions
  - (i) Purpose
  - (ii) Scope
  - (iii) Situation Overview
    - (a) Hazard Analysis Summary
    - (b) Capability Assessment
    - (c) Mitigation Overview
  - (iv) Planning Assumptions
- c) Concept of Operations
- d) Organization and Assignment of Responsibilities
- e) Direction, Control, and Coordination
- f) Information Collection, Analysis, and Dissemination
- g) Communications
- h) Administration, Finance, and Logistics
- i) Plan Development and Maintenance
- j) Authorities and References

❷ Functional Annexes

(Note: This is not a complete list. Each jurisdiction's support functions will vary.)

- a) Direction, Control, and Coordination
- b) Continuity of Government/ Operations
- c) Communications
- d) Transportation
- e) Warning
- f) External Affairs/Emergency Public Information

- g) Population Protection
- h) Mass Care, Emergency Assistance, Housing, and Human Services
- i) Public Health and Medical Services
- j) Resource Management
- k) CIKR Restoration
- l) Damage Assessment
- m) Firefighting
- n) Logistics Management and Resource Support
- o) Search and Rescue
- p) Oil and Hazardous Materials Response
- q) Agriculture and Natural Resources
- r) Energy
- s) Public Safety and Security
- t) Long-Term Community Recovery
- u) Financial Management
- v) Mutual Aid/Multi-Jurisdictional Coordination
- w) Private Sector Coordination
- x) Volunteer and Donations Management
- y) Worker Safety and Health
- z) Prevention and Protection

❸ Hazard-, Threat-, or Incident-Specific Annexes

(Note: This is not a complete list. Each jurisdiction's annexes will vary based on their hazard analysis.)

- a) Hurricane/Severe Storm
- b) Earthquake
- c) Tornado
- d) Flood/Dam Failure
- e) Hazardous Materials Incident
- f) Radiological Incident
- g) Biological Incident
- h) Terrorism Incident

FIGURE 7-4 Traditional EOP format

Data from Federal Emergency Management Agency. Developing and Maintaining Emergency Operations Plans. Comprehensive Preparedness Guide (CPG) 101. Version 2.0. Available at: www.fema.gov/media-library/assets/documents/25975. Published November 2010. Accessed August 30, 2017.

EMERGENCY SUPPORT FUNCTION EOP FORMAT

① Basic Plan

  a) Introductory Material
    (i) Promulgation Document/ Signatures
    (ii) Approval and Implementation
    (iii) Record of Changes
    (iv) Record of Distribution
    (v) Table of Contents
  b) Purpose, Scope, Situation Overview, and Assumptions
    (i) Purpose
    (ii) Scope
    (iii) Situation Overview
      (a) Hazard Analysis Summary
      (b) Capability Assessment
      (c) Mitigation Overview
    (iv) Planning Assumptions
  c) Concept of Operations
  d) Organization and Assignment of Responsibilities
  e) Direction, Control, and Coordination
  f) Information Collection, Analysis, and Dissemination
  g) Communications
  h) Administration, Finance, and Logistics
  i) Plan Development and Maintenance
  j) Authorities and References

② Emergency Support Function Annexes

  a) ESF #l – Transportation
  b) ESF #2 – Communications
  c) ESF #3 – Public Works and Engineering
  d) ESF #4 – Firefighting
  e) ESF #5 – Emergency Management
  f) ESF #6 – Mass Care, Emergency Assistance, Housing, and Human Services
  g) ESF #7 – Logistics Management and Resource Support
  h) ESF #8 – Public Health and Medical Services
  i) ESF #9 – Search and Rescue
  j) ESF #10 – Oil and Hazardous Materials Response
  k) ESF #11 – Agriculture and Natural Resources
  l) ESF #12 – Energy
  m) ESF #13 – Public Safety and Security
  n) ESF #14 – Long-Term Community Recovery
  o) ESF #15 – External Affairs
  p) Other ESFs as defined by the jurisdiction

③ Support Annexes

(Note: This is not a complete list. Each jurisdiction's support functions will vary.)

  a) Continuity of Government/ Operations
  b) Warning
  c) Population Protection
  d) Financial Management
  e) Mutual Aid/Multijurisdictional Coordination
  f) Private Sector Coordination
  g) Volunteer and Donations Management
  h) Worker Safety and Health
  i) Prevention and Protection

④ Hazard-, Threat-, or Incident-Specific Annexes

(Note: This is not a complete list. Each jurisdiction's annexes will vary based on their hazard analysis.)

  a) Hurricane/Severe Storm
  b) Earthquake
  c) Tornado
  d) Flood/Dam Failure
  e) Hazardous Materials Incident
  f) Radiological Incident
  g) Biological Incident
  h) Terrorism Incident

FIGURE 7-5 ESF format

Data from Federal Emergency Management Agency. Developing and Maintaining Emergency Operations Plans. Comprehensive Preparedness Guide (CPG) 101. Version 2.0. Available at: www.fema.gov/media-library/assets/documents/25975. Published November 2010. Accessed August 30, 2017.

AGENCY-/DEPARTMENT-FOCUSED EOP FORMAT

❶ Basic Plan

   a) Introductory Material
      (i) Promulgation Document/
         Signatures
      (ii) Approval and
         Implementation
      (iii) Record of Changes
      (iv) Record of Distribution
      (v) Table of Contents
   b) Purpose, Scope, Situation
      Overview, and Assumptions
      (i) Purpose
      (ii) Scope
      (iii) Situation Overview
         (a) Hazard Analysis
            Summary
         (b) Capability Assessment
         (c) Mitigation Overview
      (iv) Planning Assumptions
   c) Concept of Operations
   d) Organization and Assignment
      of Responsibilities
   e) Direction, Control, and
      Coordination
   f) Information Collection,
      Analysis, and Dissemination
   g) Communications
   h) Administration, Finance, and
      Logistics
   i) Plan Development and
      Maintenance
   j) Authorities and References

❷ Lead Agencies

   a) Fire
   b) Law Enforcement
   c) Emergency Medical
   d) Emergency Management
   e) Hospital
   f) Public Health
   g) Others as Needed

❸ Support Annexes

Identify those agencies that have a support role during an emergency and describe/address the strategies they are responsible for implementing.

❹ Hazard-Specific Procedures

For any response or support agency, describe/address its hazard-specific strategies.

FIGURE 7-6 Agency-focused EOP format

Data from Federal Emergency Management Agency. Developing and Maintaining Emergency Operations Plans. Comprehensive Preparedness Guide (CPG) 101. Version 2.0. Available at: www.fema.gov/media-library/assets/documents/25975. Published November 2010. Accessed August 30, 2017.

In 2007, a National Continuity Policy was issued as National Security Presidential Directive-51 (NSPD-51)/Homeland Security Presidential Directive-20 (HSPD-20). It outlined continuity requirements for all executive departments and agencies; provided guidance for states, territories, tribal areas, and local public and private entities; and designated the Secretary of Homeland Security as the leader for all continuity initiatives.[11] It is meant to ensure the performance of the eight National Essential Functions:

1. Ensuring the continued functioning of our form of government under the Constitution, including the functioning of three separate branches of government
2. Providing leadership visible to the Nation and the world and maintaining the trust and confidence of the American people
3. Defending the Constitution of the United States against all enemies, foreign and domestic, and preventing or interdicting attacks against the United States or its people, property, or interests
4. Maintaining and fostering effective relationships with foreign nations
5. Protecting against threats to the homeland and bringing to justice perpetrators of crimes or attacks against the United States or its people, property, or interests
6. Providing rapid and effective response to and recovery from the domestic consequences of an attack or other incident
7. Protecting and stabilizing the Nation's economy and ensuring public confidence in its financial systems
8. Providing for critical federal government services that address the national health, safety, and welfare needs of the United States

▶ Human Capital Risks

In the event of an emergency, human capital is the most valuable asset that an organization has. Organizations must plan to safeguard and support employees—including those who have themselves been affected by the disaster—while continuing to deliver the services needed to keep the business operational and revenue flowing. The following factors are important to consider in the human capital element of a COOP.

Employee Health

COOPs should account for employee attendance due to health and safety concerns during a disaster. Even employees who are not directly affected by a disaster may need to miss work to look after the health and safety of family members who are affected. Employees willing and able to work through a crisis may simply not be able to get to their work location because of disrupted public transportation systems or travel restrictions. Even smaller-scale disasters, such as transit system strikes and blizzards, can significantly impact employees' ability to get to work. For these reasons, it may be necessary to consider telecommuting policies. Adopting a virtual working environment requires that organizations address specific technology and communication requirements, including providing remote access and support, online tools, and collaborative workspaces. Organizations also must closely examine their processes to better understand how they can be executed in a virtual environment.

In addition, employee shock and grief can lead to increased absenteeism, as well as higher turnover and reduced productivity. Proactive counseling may be required to help employees confront emergent issues as well as enable them to address the crisis more rapidly.

Internal Communication

Communications systems (cell phones, landlines, and other communications networks) can be destroyed or become dysfunctional in a disaster, making it difficult to locate employees and share critical information with them. Unsafe facilities or those that are inaccessible to some individuals can make it more difficult for staff to collaborate and tap into their existing social and professional networks. The inability to bring people together can significantly hamper the rapid decision-making needed during recovery efforts. Without normal communication channels, maintaining business relationships with customers and business partners will also be difficult.

Payroll and Human Resources

Maintaining payroll is both essential and challenging during and following a crisis. Inaccessible payroll systems, limited funds, or the absence of payroll staff will make it difficult to pay employees in a timely manner. Employees may also need disaster relief funding, which requires coordination from a variety of sources.

Human resources departments should plan to deliver other core services during a crisis, as well as to monitor and report on the locations of displaced workers. Third-party providers who have been hired to manage these processes should also be prepared to deal with emergencies.

Employee Tracking

Employee tracking can affect an organization's ability to resume operations after a crisis. This includes limited access to critical personnel data, such as emergency contact information, user IDs and passwords, and a database of individual skill sets. Furthermore, the inability of an organization to determine which employees have been impacted by the crisis will make it difficult for decision makers to determine the organization's next steps. Recovery efforts can be further hampered if an organization cannot locate key personnel or access core business systems, or has not identified or arranged for potential replacement workers.

Succession Planning

During or after a crisis, organizational leaders could be incapacitated or unavailable. If an organization has not engaged in formal succession planning, individuals at all levels may be forced to take on leadership roles or increased responsibilities with little or no preparation. Staffing issues can also emerge as a reduced workforce tries to cope with the demands of an increased workload. Skill gaps can also become a problem as workers try to carry out changes in employee locations and schedules that are difficult to keep track of in a fast-changing environment.

To mitigate these risks, it is important to cross-train employees on key skills and capabilities so they can take on new responsibilities, if needed. Foster mentoring between individuals where experiential knowledge is critical and hard to capture, and initiate job shadowing as an effective technique for building redundant skills between employees.

▶ Centers for Disease Control and Prevention National Capabilities and Assistant Secretary for Preparedness and Response Capabilities

To help state and local public health departments strategically plan for emergencies and disasters, the Centers for Disease Control and Prevention (CDC) developed capabilities as national standards.[12] Similarly, the U.S. Department of Health and Human Services, Office of the Assistant Secretary for Preparedness and Response (ASPR) identified eight capabilities for healthcare systems to develop[13] as key to their role in emergency preparedness and response. Eight CDC capabilities correspond to the ASPR measures for healthcare system preparedness. The CDC's National Capability Standards are:

1. **Community Preparedness:** The ability of communities to prepare for, withstand, and recover from—in both the short and long terms—public health incidents. *Aligned ASPR Capability: Healthcare System Preparedness.*

2. **Community Recovery:** The ability to collaborate with community partners (such as healthcare organizations, businesses, and emergency management) to plan and advocate for the rebuilding of public health, medical, and mental/behavioral health systems to at least a level of functioning comparable to pre-incident levels, and improved levels where possible. *Aligned ASPR Capability: Healthcare System Recovery.*

3. **Emergency Operations Coordination:** The ability to direct and support an event or incident with public health or medical implications by establishing a standardized, scalable system of oversight, organization, and supervision consistent with jurisdictional standards and practices and with the NIMS. *Aligned ASPR Capability: Emergency Operations Coordination.*

4. **Emergency Public Information and Warning:** The ability to develop, coordinate, and disseminate information, alerts, warnings, and notifications to the public and incident management responders.

5. **Fatality Management:** The ability to coordinate with other organizations (such as law enforcement, healthcare, emergency management, and medical examiners) to ensure the proper recovery, handling, identification, transportation, tracking, storage, and disposal of human remains and personal effects; certify cause of death; and facilitate access to mental/behavioral health services to the family members, responders, and survivors of an incident. *Aligned ASPR Capability: Fatality Management.*

6. **Information Sharing:** The ability to conduct multijurisdictional, multidisciplinary exchange of health-related information and situational awareness data among federal, state, local, territorial, and tribal levels of government, and the private sector. *Aligned ASPR Capability: Information Sharing.*

7. **Mass Care:** The ability to coordinate with partner agencies to address the public health, medical, and mental/behavioral health needs of those impacted by an incident at a congregate location.

8. **Medical Countermeasure Dispensing:** The ability to provide medical countermeasures (including vaccines, antiviral drugs, antibiotics, antitoxins, etc.) in support of treatment or prophylaxis (oral or vaccination) to the identified population in accordance with public health guidelines and/or recommendations.

9. **Medical Materiel Management and Distribution:** The ability to acquire, maintain (through cold-chain storage or other storage protocol), transport, distribute, and track medical materiel (such as pharmaceuticals, gloves, masks and ventilators) during an incident and to recover and account for unused medical materiel, as necessary, after an incident.

10. **Medical Surge:** The ability to provide adequate medical evaluation and care during events that exceed the limits of the normal medical infrastructure of an affected community. *Aligned ASPR Capability: Medical Surge.*

11. **Nonpharmaceutical Interventions:** The ability to recommend to the applicable lead agency (if not public health) and implement, if applicable, strategies for disease, injury, and exposure control.

12. **Public Health Laboratory Testing:** The ability to conduct rapid and conventional detection, characterization, confirmatory testing, data reporting, investigative support, and laboratory networking to address actual or potential exposure to all hazards.

13. **Public Health Surveillance and Epidemiological Investigation:** The ability to create, maintain, support, and strengthen routine surveillance and detection systems and epidemiological investigation processes, as well as to expand these systems and processes in response to incidents of public health significance.

14. **Responder Safety and Health:** The ability to protect public health agency staff responding to an incident and the ability to support the health and safety needs of hospital and medical facility personnel, if requested. *Aligned ASPR Capability: Responder Safety and Health.*

15. **Volunteer Management:** The ability to coordinate the identification, recruitment, registration, credential verification, training, and engagement of volunteers to support the jurisdictional public health agency's response to incidents of public health significance. *Aligned ASPR Capability: Volunteer Management.*

As public health departments develop preparedness plans, they should do so with an eye toward developing (and practicing, as we see in Chapter 8) these capabilities.

Partnerships and Coalition Building

The work of preparing for, preventing, responding to, and recovering from emergencies cannot be done by government alone. Even in smaller-scale disasters, which government agencies are generally effective at managing, service gaps still exist. Due to the effects of climate change, the severity and frequency of certain disasters are growing and will pose increasingly greater threats.[14]

To be effective, preparedness activities must take a "whole community" approach in which government agencies and officials work jointly with healthcare systems, community leaders, humanitarian organizations, faith-based organizations, schools, private businesses, and individuals. As is commonly said, an emergency is not the time to be passing out business cards; fruitful partnerships and relationships must be established in advance so that when an emergency occurs, all parties can carry out their roles and responsibilities. Accordingly, the roles and responsibilities of each part of the community must be reflected in all preparedness plans and materials.

In developing the whole-community philosophy, FEMA developed six strategic themes that describe how to apply this philosophy in emergency management preparedness planning. These themes are as follows:

1. **Understand community complexity.** Get a clear understanding of local populations, how they interact and organize, their typical needs, and how those needs are typically met under normal (nonemergency) circumstances. What are its demographics, values, and existing networks?

2. **Recognize community capabilities and needs.** Understand what the community's needs and capabilities would be in an emergency, including how they can contribute to improved outcomes.

3. **Foster relationships with community leaders.** Look to trusted formal and informal community leaders to help identify a community's interests and receptiveness to preparedness campaigns. Build relationships of trust over time.

4. **Build and maintain partnerships.** Form and nurture multiorganizational partnerships to ensure that a wide variety of community interests are represented in preparedness planning.

5. **Empower local action.** Let community members take the lead in identifying their own priorities, organizing support around those priorities, implementing programs, and evaluating program effectiveness.

6. **Leverage and strengthen social infrastructure, networks, and assets.** Invest in the systems that already define daily life in a community and align emergency management activities to those systems.

▶ Conclusion

All communities are subject to hazards. Hazards can occur due to natural forces, such as weather patterns and occurrences, or due to human forces, such as acts of terrorism. The Preparedness Cycle provides the framework through which emergency planners build capability and capacity for response to these threats, first by assessing the hazards to which their communities are most susceptible, then developing plans to address each hazard, training staff on the implementation of emergency response plans, and finally conducting drills and exercises to test the viability of the plans.

In addition to hazard-specific response plans, other plans are often necessary to ensure that organizations continue to operate properly, even in the midst of an emergency. COOPs outline the processes that organizations, particularly government organizations, will use to discontinue nonessential services during emergencies, while maintaining essential services and caring for the organization's resources and assets.

In emergency preparedness and response, the importance of partnerships and coalitions cannot be overemphasized. Government entities continue to be grossly under-resourced, but their capability can be augmented by community and private-sector resources. Recognizing the need for and establishing relationships with nontraditional response partners, during peace time, can provide significant capability for emergency response, despite resource scarcity. The ability of a community to remain resilient following the occurrence of a disaster can be facilitated through these partnerships as well as a "whole community" approach to preparedness. Planning that includes all voices of a community can be a significant factor in how quickly and fairly people return to work, school, worship, and play.

Discussion Questions

1. Name and define each component of the preparedness cycle.
2. What is an HVA, and why is conducting this assessment so important to preparedness?
3. What is a RNA? Why is the RNA completed *after* the occurrence of an emergency event?
4. What are three different formats for EOPs? Which format would be most appropriate to use when planning for a specific agency's role in support of a larger emergency response effort?
5. What is the whole-of-community approach to preparedness? Which specific piece of legislation calls for the whole-of-community approach? Describe a recent emergency event where the whole-of-community approach was utilized to ensure proper response to the event.

References

1. Department of Homeland Security. Plan and prepare for disasters. Available at https://www.dhs.gov/topic/plan-and-prepare-disasters. Published June 23, 2017. Accessed August 29, 2017.
2. Federal Emergency Management Agency. Preparedness cycle. Available at https://www.fema.gov/media-library/assets/images/114295#. Accessed August 29, 2017.
3. U.S. Department of Health and Human Services. MSCC: the healthcare coalition in emergency response and recovery. Available at https://www.phe.gov/Preparedness/planning/mscc/Documents/mscctier2jan2010.pdf. Reviewed August 25, 2010. Accessed August 29, 2017.
4. Federal Emergency Management Agency. Hazard identification and risk assessment. Available at https://www.fema.gov/hazard-identification-and-risk-assessment. Updated August 4, 2017. Accessed August 29, 2017.
5. Department of Homeland Security. Risk assessment. Available at https://www.ready.gov/risk-assessment. Accessed August 28, 2017.
6. Federal Emergency Management Agency. National preparedness goal core capabilities. Available at https://www.fema.gov/core-capabilities. Updated July 25, 2017. Accessed August 29, 2017.
7. Federal Emergency Management Agency. *Threat and Hazard Identification Risk Assessment Guide. Comprehensive Preparedness Guide (CPG) 201.* 2nd ed. Available at https://www.fema.gov/media-library-data/20130726-1831-250450138/cpg_201_supp_1_thira_guide_toolkit_final_040312.pdf. Published August 2013. Accessed August 29, 2017.
8. Federal Emergency Management Agency. *Developing and Maintaining Emergency Operations Plans. Comprehensive Preparedness Guide (CPG) 101.* Version 2.0. Available at https://www.fema.gov/media-library/assets/documents/25975. Published November 2010. Accessed August 30, 2017.

9. FEMA. Policy, plans and evaluation division. Available at https://www.fema.gov/policy-plans-evaluations.
10. U.S. Department of Health and Human Services, Centers for Disease Control and Prevention. Public health preparedness capabilities: national standards for capability development. https://www.cdc.gov/phpr/readiness/00_docs/DSLR_capabilities_July.pdf. Accessed August 30, 2017.
11. https://www.fema.gov/pdf/about/org/ncp/nspd_51.pdf. Accessed August 30, 2017.
12. U.S. Centers for Disease Control. Public health preparedness capabilities: national standards for state and local planning. Available at https://www.cdc.gov/phpr/readiness/00_docs/DSLR_capabilities_July.pdf. Published March 2011. Accessed August 29, 2017.
13. U.S. Department of Health and Human Services. Healthcare preparedness capabilities: national guidance for healthcare system preparedness. Available at https://www.phe.gov/preparedness/planning/hpp/reports/documents/capabilities.pdf.
14. Intergovernmental Panel on Climate Change. Special report on managing the risks of extreme events and disasters to advance climate change adaptation. May 2012.

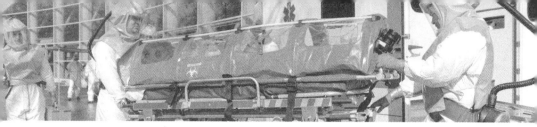

CHAPTER 8

Training, Exercising, and Evaluating

LEARNING OBJECTIVES

After assessment and planning, the remainder of the preparedness cycle focuses on putting plans into practice and evaluating the results, always with an eye toward continuous improvement. Training, exercising, and evaluating are never-ending processes that must continually adapt to changing circumstances, changing staff, and new information. By the end of this chapter, readers should be able to:

- Understand how training, exercising, and evaluating complete the preparedness cycle, and how the cycle resets
- Understand the goal of exercises and articulate the various types of exercises
- Explain the Homeland Security Exercise and Evaluation Program (HSEEP) methodology
- Explain how the use of after action reports (AARs) and improvement plans (IPs) contributes to increased preparedness

▶ Introduction

Training has always been an important part of the public health infrastructure. Assuring a competent workforce is one of the Ten Essential Public Health Services, part of the Assurance function. That said, in the years following September 11, 2001 (9/11), there was a heightened focus on training for emergency preparedness, with significant federal funds allocated for this purpose. Skills in planning, communications, surveillance, management, and leadership were essential not only within organizations but also across sectors within communities. The HSEEP program provided a framework for organizing activities in training, exercising, and evaluating that in effect has become an all-hazards approach for preparedness training.

▶ Training

Emergency preparedness training is aimed at increasing the competence of public health workers to prevent, prepare for, respond to, and recover from public health emergencies. Training is generally conducted to ensure the skills needed to execute emergency response plans and build public health capability are achieved. For example, if an emergency operations plan includes establishing a mobile command center in a tent, responders would need to be trained on how to set up the tent, what equipment and supplies are needed to operate the tent, and what the ideal location within the tent should be for each piece of equipment for maximum operational efficiency.

Most of the core competencies that emergency preparedness officials are required to meet come from four primary sources:

- Foundational public health competencies, such as the Council on Linkages Between Academia and Public Health Practice Core Competencies for Public Health Professionals[1] and the Association of Schools and Programs of Public Health (ASPPH) Master's Degree in Public Health Core Competency Model[2] for those in the target group with specific training in public health
- Health security or emergency management core competencies, such as those that may stem from National Incident Management System (NIMS) courses or competency sets developed by the Federal Emergency Management Agency's (FEMA) Emergency Management Institute[3]
- Position- or capability-specific competencies, as outlined in the Centers for Disease Control and Prevention (CDC) Public Health Preparedness Capabilities: National Standards for State and Local Planning[4]

The CDC and the ASPPH developed the Public Health Preparedness and Response Competency Map to provide a national competency-based training to measure preparedness and response capability. It represents all core competencies that public health workers are expected to demonstrate to ensure readiness. **FIGURE 8-1** shows a graphical representation of the model.

▶ Exercising

Once emergency preparedness personnel have been trained on their roles and responsibilities during an emergency, a series of increasingly complex exercises in a low-risk environment helps reinforce learning, test capabilities, improve performance, and validate plans—or expose plan shortcomings that must be addressed. Exercises are an opportunity for personnel to practice all policies, plans, and procedures; use equipment that will be required during an incident; rehearse communications procedures within and among organizations; and practice coordinating decision making. Exercises also serve as a means "to bring together and strengthen participants under the "whole community" approach to prevent, protect against, mitigate, respond to, and recover from all hazards."[5]

The HSEEP was developed to provide a set of guiding principles for exercise programs and a common framework for planning and conducting various types of exercises. This methodology, released in 2013, gives jurisdictions a consistent approach to designing, conducting, and evaluating exercises, and ultimately, improving plans based on post exercise findings. **FIGURE 8-2** illustrates the exercise

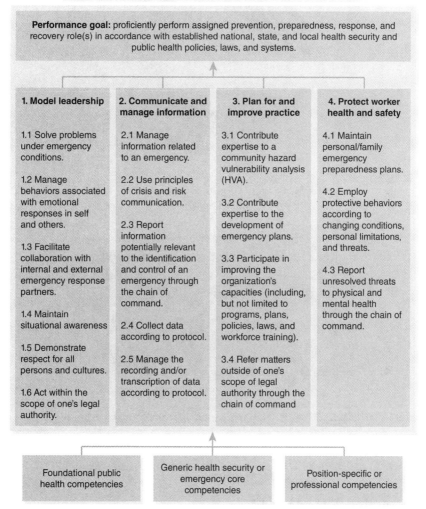

Public health preparedness and response competency map
(model version 1.0 - December 14, 2010)

Performance goal: proficiently perform assigned prevention, preparedness, response, and recovery role(s) in accordance with established national, state, and local health security and public health policies, laws, and systems.

1. Model leadership	2. Communicate and manage information	3. Plan for and improve practice	4. Protect worker health and safety
1.1 Solve problems under emergency conditions.	2.1 Manage information related to an emergency.	3.1 Contribute expertise to a community hazard vulnerability analysis (HVA).	4.1 Maintain personal/family emergency preparedness plans.
1.2 Manage behaviors associated with emotional responses in self and others.	2.2 Use principles of crisis and risk communication.	3.2 Contribute expertise to the development of emergency plans.	4.2 Employ protective behaviors according to changing conditions, personal limitations, and threats.
1.3 Facilitate collaboration with internal and external emergency response partners.	2.3 Report information potentially relevant to the identification and control of an emergency through the chain of command.	3.3 Participate in improving the organization's capacities (including, but not limited to programs, plans, policies, laws, and workforce training).	4.3 Report unresolved threats to physical and mental health through the chain of command.
1.4 Maintain situational awareness	2.4 Collect data according to protocol.		
1.5 Demonstrate respect for all persons and cultures.	2.5 Manage the recording and/or transcription of data according to protocol.	3.4 Refer matters outside of one's scope of legal authority through the chain of command	
1.6 Act within the scope of one's legal authority.			

Foundational public health competencies	Generic health security or emergency core competencies	Position-specific or professional competencies

This project is conducted in partnership under a cooperative agreement between CDC and ASPH.

FIGURE 8-1 Public health preparedness and response competency map. December 14, 2010

Data from Centers for Disease Control and Prevention and Association of Schools of Public Health. Public Health Preparedness & Response Model. Available at: www.aspph.org/teach-research/models/public-health-preparedness-response/ Accessed: August 26, 2017.

cycle. The program summarizes much of the timing, logistical, and methodological issues involved in creating exercises. It also demonstrates how to establish links between evaluation operations and testable, measurable outcomes.[5]

Under HSEEP, exercises are progressive and utilize a building-block approach that spans multiple years. The program defines two broad categories: discussion-based exercises and operations-based exercises. **FIGURE 8-3** shows the progression through the types of activities toward increasing capability. Eventually, by drilling in situations that are as close to real-world conditions as possible, all participants will be better prepared to perform under the stressful, often chaotic conditions of an actual disaster.

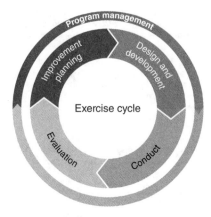

FIGURE 8-2 HSEEP exercise cycle

Data from U.S. Department of Homeland Security, Homeland Security Exercise and Evaluation Program. Available at: www.fema.gov
/media-library-data/20130726-1914-25045-8890/hseep_apr13_.pdf. Published April 2013. Accessed August 26, 2017.

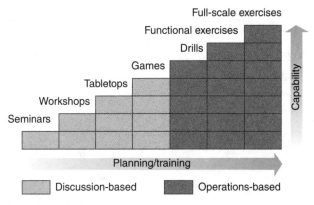

FIGURE 8-3 The building block approach

Data from FEMA, EMI Course: IS-120.a. An Introduction to Exercises Available at: www.training.fema.gov/is/courseoverview
.aspx?code=IS-120.a. Accessed: August 26, 2017.

Discussion-Based Exercises

Discussion-bases exercises, such as seminars, workshops, tabletop exercises, and simu-
lations, provide a forum for discussing or developing plans, agreements, trainings, and
procedures. They "focus on strategic and policy-level issues"[5], are less complicated than
operations-based exercises, and do not involve the actual deployment of resources.
Exercises at the discussion level are more theory than practice. The four types of
discussion-based exercises are seminars, workshops, tabletop exercises, and games.

Seminars

During seminars, participants will review plans and become familiar with plans
from agency and jurisdiction partners. The goal of a seminar is to introduce or rein-
troduce participants to plans and assess partner capabilities. Seminars are casual in
nature and can be relatively informal.

Workshops

Workshops involve a more formal, hands-on approach to developing, modifying, and learning plans. Workshops are collaborative in nature and encourage open discussion, brainstorming, information sharing, and consensus building. Breakout sessions can give smaller groups a chance to explore issues in more depth. In a situation where an emergency plan needs to be developed or revised, a workshop can be used to drive this process.

Tabletop

During tabletop exercises, participants and partners can talk through the execution of plans to identify strengths and areas for improvement. These exercises can be somewhat informal in nature and typically involve senior staff or officials discussing plans in the context of hypothetical emergencies. These discussions can expose shortcomings in a plan and provide an open forum in which leaders can collaboratively work toward solutions.

Games

Games are simulated exercises of increasing complexity that give participants a chance to test plans against various "what if?" scenarios. While games do not involve the use of actual resources, they are highly useful for testing ideas and decision-making processes to improve participants' understanding.

Operations-Based Exercises

Operations-based exercises entail the execution of plans, policies, and procedures. They are more complex and involve the actual deployment of resources to test plans against real-world conditions. The goals of operations-based exercises are to give participants a chance to practice their roles and responsibilities, "identify resource gaps"[5], and raise the performance level of all teams and participants. The three types of operations-based exercises are drills, functional exercises, and full-scale exercises.

Drills

Drills typically are supervised activities designed to test a single, specific operation within a single organization. For example, in a drill, an SWAT team might conduct an active shooter drill. The main goals of a drill are to train participants on any new equipment they may need to use and to test the procedures created in the planning stage. Drills are relatively realistic, but they are conducted in contained environments. They are useful for generating real-time feedback on the quality of a team's preparedness and capabilities and helping participants prepare for more complex exercises in the future.

Functional Exercises

Functional exercises are typically conducted to evaluate an agency's ability to carry out multiple functions or to assess the coordination between various responding agencies. For example, a public health department may conduct a functional exercise for activating a medication dispensing center to get experience setting up the layout of the location, installing the necessary equipment, and establishing the flow of patients through the center. Functional exercises require on-the-spot problem solving and can be relatively high-stress situations.

Full-Scale Exercises

Full-scale exercises are the most complex and realistic category of preparedness exercises. They are multiagency, multijurisdictional, and multidisciplinary events to test the full depth and breadth of an emergency response. For example, multiple city agencies may run a full-scale exercise to test the response to an outbreak of a highly infectious disease. Full-scale exercises involve the actual deployment of resources and are meant to be as realistic as possible. As such, they can be highly stressful but are an extremely useful final step in testing and validating all aspects of a response plan.

▶ Evaluation

The goal of conducting exercises is to evaluate their effectiveness and respond accordingly. Evaluation of preparedness activities "involves the systematic collection of information that assists stakeholders to better understand a program, improve its effectiveness, and make decisions about future programming".[6] In general, an evaluation should determine the strengths and weakness of the response and whether it meets the intended needs, audiences, and measurable objectives. Another important purpose of an exercise evaluation is to use data gathered from observation that will reduce morbidity and mortality during a disaster. Insight gleaned from an evaluation may also result in adjustments to plans for efficiency, improved response efforts, and cost-effectiveness.[7]

Evaluation Design

Effective evaluation design begins in the planning stages with the establishment of measurable objectives and determination of indicators. The plan should also delineate the processes for conducting an evaluation, including personnel and duties, coordination, and oversight. The five tasks typically associated with planning an evaluation are:

- "Selecting a lead evaluator and defin[ing] evaluation team requirements
- Developing Exercise Evaluation Guides (EEGs), which include objectives, core capabilities, capability targets and critical tasks
- Recruiting, training and assigning evaluators
- Developing and finalizing evaluation documentation
- Conducting a pre-exercise controller/evaluator briefing"[5(p5-1)]

Evaluation Team

A lead evaluator will oversee the evaluation process and will work with the team to determine the structure of the team, objectives, and all tasks that will be evaluated. The lead evaluator is also responsible for deciding which data collection methods will be used and how data will be recorded.

Developing Exercise Evaluation Guides (EEGs)

EEGs are a tool to guide the evaluator's work as they observe exercises and collect data. These guides should streamline the collection of data, be aligned with capability targets, support the development of an AAR, assess preparedness consistently through all exercises, and help map results to objectives, capabilities, targets, and next steps for improvement.[5(pp5-2–5-3)]

Recruiting, Assigning, and Training Evaluators

The lead evaluator determines how many evaluators are necessary, what subject matter expertise is required, and whether evaluators will require any training prior to the evaluation.

Developing and Finalizing Evaluation Documentation

The lead evaluator is responsible for compiling all documentation, including a C/E handbook or evaluation plan that addresses:

- "Exercise-specific details: the scenario being exercised and the schedule of events
- Evaluator team details: the team structure, locations, shift assignments, maps and contact information
- Evaluator instructions: a step-by-step set of instructions for evaluators to follow before, during and after the exercise
- Evaluation tools: EEGs, electronic or manual evaluation logs, participant feedback forms and templates for After-Action Reports"[5(pp5–3)]

Evaluation Methods

Objective review of a disaster plan throughout the different stages in its development and execution provides information on how to improve the plan to meet the demands of a given disaster scenario in the future. Evaluators revise programs by determining the objectives of the disaster plan, identifying appropriate measures for each objective, and collecting data to substantiate that those objectives are met during the execution of the exercise. This is meant to be an ongoing cycle of review and improvement.

Domains of Activity

"Evaluations assess five domains of activity:

1. Structure. Are exercises structured in such a way that they simulate the type of hazard the plan is designed to address?
2. Process. Is the process for executing the tasks clearly defined and are those tasks being executed according to the process?
3. Outcomes. Do outcomes align with the expectations? If not, what areas fall short?
4. Response adequacy. Does the response follow a logical progression that addresses the hazard?
5. Costs. Are there additional costs that have not been anticipated in the plan?[5]"

Data Collection

Data should be collected throughout the planning, impact, and postimpact phases of a disaster. During exercises, evaluators should collect data in many forms and from many sources, including epidemiological data, media reports, environmental and medical assessments, and interviews, real or simulated. It is critical that evaluators retain their notes and records, because those items will be used in the next step: developing the AAR.

The lead evaluator may assign evaluators to collect additional data during or immediately after the exercise. For example, useful sources of supplemental evaluation data might include records produced by automated systems or communication networks, and written records, such as duty logs and message forms.[5]

After Action Reports (AARs)

Immediately after the conclusion of an exercise, evaluators should begin the task of creating AARs, which are summary reports that highlight any lessons learned and provide all exercise participants with general and specific feedback on the exercise. The main focus of this report should be on core capabilities and the response team's performance related to stated objectives. Were capability targets met? If not, why not? What caused the response to fall short of its stated goal? The AAR should also identify all strengths, weaknesses, and potential areas for improvement. These issues should then be taken into account in future planning and exercises. These "lessons learned" from the AAR process can be used to build upon the experiences of the exercise participants.[8] This information is useful to improve the conduct and execution of future planning and exercise activities. AARs should be shared with any collaborating partners as necessary.

Improvement Plans

After completion of the AAR, leaders examine the reports to determine whether the conclusions drawn are valid and require corrective action. Once leaders reach consensus on this question, organizations must convert AAR recommendations into steps that participants can use to improve preparedness and response capabilities in the future. IPs must include specific and measurable objectives outline particular improvement tasks for designated roles or agencies, and establish a timeline for completion of those tasks.[5]

▶ Conclusion

Training, exercising, and evaluating are the final components of the preparedness cycle. After the assessment and planning phases have been executed, emergency responders must be trained on the skills and competencies they will need to conduct their responsibilities within the plan. Training gives emergency responders an understanding of what their roles will be and the importance of those roles. Following training, exercises are conducted to provide real or simulated experiences that mimic actual emergencies. This gives emergency responders the opportunity to put their training to work. Exercises can be discussion-based or operations-based, and should provide the participants with an experience that is as close to reality as possible. Incorporating logistical, financial, and operational details contributes to the real-world context. The HSEEP program is designed to help jurisdictions address many of the timing, logistic, budgetary, and methodological issues involved in creating any kind of testing exercise. It also demonstrates how to build links between exercise evaluation and testable, measurable outcomes.

Data collection and evaluation of exercises provide valuable information that can be used to improve the plans and the response actions they are designed to address. Sustaining this training, exercise, and evaluation cycle over time is an important part of public health practice at the local, state, and regional levels.

Discussion Questions

1. What is the relationship between training, exercises, and evaluation to the assessment and planning phases of the preparedness cycle?
2. What is HSEEP? How does the HSEEP methodology assist emergency workers in gaining skill in executing their preparedness roles?
3. What are the two main types of exercises? Describe at least one major difference in each type, and explain how that difference contributes to the value of the exercise.
4. How does the use of AARs and IPs contribute to increased preparedness?

References

1. Public Health Foundation. Council on linkages between academia and public health. Core Competencies for Public Health Professionals. Available at http://www.phf.org/programs /council/Pages/default.aspx/CCs-example-free-ADOPTED.pdf and http://www.phf.org/resources tools/Documents/Core_Competencies_for_Public_Health_Professionals_2014June.pdf. (Core Competencies; Published June 26, 2014.) Accessed August 26, 2017.
2. Association of Schools and Programs of Public Health. Master's degree in public health core competency development project. Available at http://www.aspph.org/app/uploads /2014/04/Version2.31_FINAL.pdf. Published August 2006. Accessed August 26, 2017.
3. FEMA. Emergency Management Institute. Available at https://training.fema.gov/emi.aspx. Accessed August 26, 2017.
4. Centers for Disease Control and Prevention. Public health preparedness capabilities: national standards for state and local planning. Available at https://www.cdc.gov/phpr /readiness/00_docs/DSLR_capabilities_July.pdf. Published March 2011. Accessed August 26, 2017.
5. U.S. Department of Homeland Security. Homeland security exercise and evaluation program. Available at https://www.fema.gov/media-library-data/20130726-1914-25045-8890/hseep _apr13_.pdf. Published April 2013. Accessed August 26, 2017.
6. US Army Public Health Command. Public health assessment & program evaluation. Available at http://phc.amedd.army.mil/topics/healthsurv/phape/Pages/default.aspx. Accessed August 29, 2017.
7. Landesman LY. *Public Health Management of Disasters: The Practice Guide.* 3rd ed. Washington, DC: APHA Press; 2011.
8. Savoia E, Agboola F, Biddinger PD. Use of after action reports (AARs) to promote organizational and systems learning in emergency preparedness. *Int J Environ Res Public Health.* 2012;9(8):2949–2963. doi:10.3390/ijerph9082949.

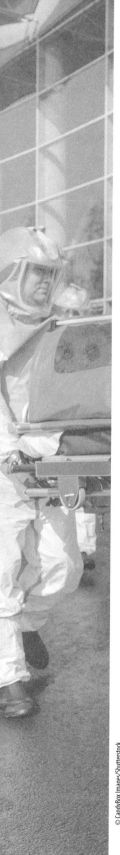

PART IV

Incident Management

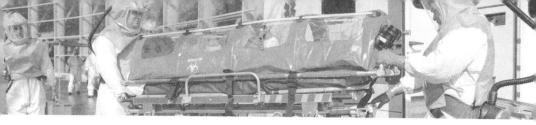

CHAPTER 9

Multiagency Coordination Systems, Information Sharing, and Interoperability

LEARNING OBJECTIVES

Emergencies require that government at all levels, the private sector, and nonprofit organizations work together to prepare for, prevent, respond to, and recover from the effects of incidents. For this to occur, there must be a framework to organize responders and coordinate their efforts. Two systems that have established the framework to improve coordination are the National Incident Management System (NIMS) and Incident Command System (ICS). NIMS is a comprehensive, national approach to incident management developed by the Federal Emergency Management Agency (FEMA) that is applicable at all jurisdictional levels and across functional disciplines and can be applied to emergencies of all types. Locally, ICS—one element of the NIMS command and management component—provides a coordinated framework for first responders to organize themselves in emergency situations. In this chapter, we take a deeper dive into NIMS and ICS and examine how these two systems help frame a larger command and management structure in incidents requiring response by multiple agencies. By the end of this chapter, readers should be able to:

- Describe NIMS and ICS
- Explain the importance of utilizing these two systems in emergency response
- Define multiagency coordination systems (MACSs) and articulate how MACSs are used in complex incident response efforts
- Explain the meaning of concepts such as common operating picture, interoperable communication, and communication redundancy

▶ National Incident Management System (NIMS)

The National Incident Management System (NIMS) is a comprehensive, national approach to incident management that is applicable at all jurisdictional levels and across functional disciplines.[1] It provides the framework for the management of incidents regardless of size, scope, or cause. Established by Homeland Security Presidential Directive 5 (HSPD-5), NIMS was designed to ensure a coordinated response to domestic disaster events and required all jurisdictions (federal, state, local, tribal, and territorial) and emergency management disciplines to comply with NIMS and utilize the unified framework for response.[1] The purpose of HSPD-5, which was issued on February 28, 2003, was to enhance the ability of the United States to manage domestic incidents by establishing a single, comprehensive national incident management system.[2] NIMS established ICS as the standard model for managing emergency events and thus ensures a common standard for overall incident management.

NIMS does not take command away from state and local authorities. The intention of the federal government is not to command the response, but rather to support state and local governments and to provide additional resources when needed. NIMS consists of five components that work together to form a comprehensive incident management system.

- Preparedness
- Communications and information management
- Resource management
- Command and management
- Ongoing management and maintenance[1]

The command and management component includes the incident command system (ICS), multiagency coordination systems (MACSs), and public information, which together facilitate incident management. See **FIGURE 9-1**.

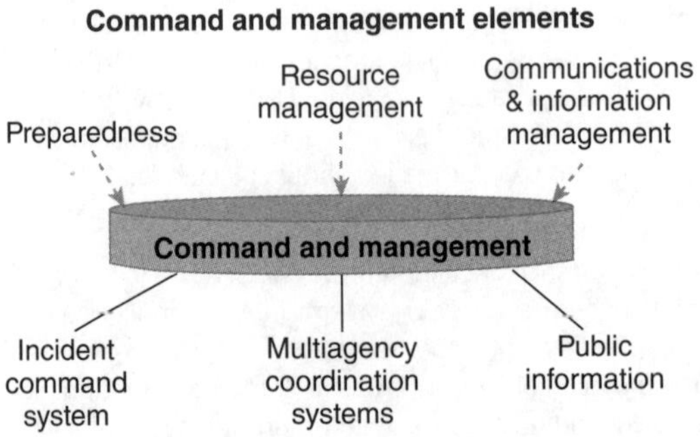

Command and management elements

Resource management
Communications & information management
Preparedness

Command and management

Incident command system
Multiagency coordination systems
Public information

FIGURE 9-1 Command and management elements

Data from Federal Emergency Management Agency, Emergency Management Institute. IS-701a. NIMS Multiagency Coordination Systems Training Course. Available at: www.training.fema.gov/is/coursematerials.aspx?code=is-701.a. Accessed June 18, 2016.

▶ Incident Command System (ICS)

When an incident requires coordination from multiple response agencies, a common set of processes and systems is critical to ensure an effective and timely response. The ICS provides a flexible, yet standardized approach for a coordinated and collaborative incident management response between agencies and across jurisdictions. Created by the National Fire Service in the early 1970s as a means to manage the response to forest fires in California, the ICS is designed to assure an organized, coordinated, rapid, and seamless response to an emergency.[3] It provides a common language, free of jargon and code words, among multiple responders, which is a major and frequent pain point in emergency response. The common and plain language mitigates the risk for miscommunication during emergencies when confusion can hamper response efforts. In addition, ICS identifies a clear chain of command and reporting structure. The system is flexible, allowing responders to meet the needs of emergencies of various scales, and cost-effective so it can also be utilized in routine operations.

ICS Structure

In the ICS structure, personnel are organized into three categories: incident commander (IC), command staff, and general staff. The IC manages and directs incident activities, directs command staff and all section chiefs, and approves ordering and releasing of resources, like medical materiel.

The command staff, including the Public Information Officer (PIO), Liaison Officer (LO), Safety Officer (SO), and Administrative Officer (AO), report directly to the IC. The PIO assures accurate and timely information to the media. The LO interacts with other partners, securing the necessary commitments and resources from other agencies. The SO manages worker safety precautions and regulations. The AO oversees the administrative component of the response, including records management.

The general staff includes the section chiefs from each of the four functional sections: Planning, Logistics, Operations, and Finance/Administration. For public health responses, a fifth functional section—Epidemiology and Surveillance, or simply Surveillance—has been included to address the threat of disease to the population. Epidemiology and Surveillance are core functions of public health, so without their integration into the model, the risk to public health would not be sufficiently addressed. In some cases, some public health departments will merely make Surveillance a component of the Planning or Operations sections, while others will designate it as a separate functional section.

The **Planning** Section has multiple responsibilities. First, Planning collects situation and resource status information to evaluate and process that information for use in developing action plans. The Planning Section documents all actions taken during the response. It feeds important information to the IC for briefings and press conferences. Additionally, this section assures staff has important information needed for carrying out assigned roles. Finally, Planning makes projections where the response should be in 24, 48, and 72 hours.

The **Logistics** Section provides all incident support needs. This entails provision of nonpersonnel resources such as securing supplies, equipment, and services for the response. Logistics also has other responsibilities, such as transporting staff and supplies, setting up phone banks, and arranging meals.

The **Operations** Section manages all tactical operations at an incident. Some of these duties include implementing response plans and managing staff, notifying and activating staff, operating points of dispensing, scheduling work, training staff, and modifying routine operations to ensure adequate staff are available for the response.

The **Finance and Administration** Section manages all financial aspects of the response, secures emergency contracts for supplies and services, tracks costs, assures staff is compensated for time worked, and seeks federal reimbursement for response-related expenditures.[3]

Finally, for public health departments, the **Surveillance** Section conducts epidemiological investigation, determines risk of exposure, identifies populations in need of prophylaxis, provides recommendations to the healthcare community and public, and determines criteria to be used for identification of cases and controls.

In an emergency, public health staff will be assigned to jobs based on their skills and experience. For example, when ICS is activated, a public health nurse working in a public health clinic would most likely be assigned to the Operations Section because the Operations Section will implement the actual response plans. Likewise, staff from facilities management would most likely be assigned to the Logistics Section, and epidemiologists and physicians to the Surveillance Section, which will perform illness investigation and disease tracking. One important change to note is that staff would report through the ICS-assigned supervisor, not to their regular supervisor.

Today, ICS is used by FEMA and other emergency management agencies throughout the United States. Hospitals, healthcare systems, and public health organizations have also adopted a form of ICS that is modified to suit their needs. ICS facilitates and improves coordination between disciplines in the public health field, improving the effectiveness and timeliness of their emergency response.

Incident Management

Incident management refers to the application of general management principles—staffing/training, planning, organizing, directing, purchasing, and monitoring—to establish and maintain relationships between all parties involved. Successful incident management is based on the recognition of diverse perspectives, and their potential impact on all phases of an emergency response. It includes the careful consideration of ethical and moral implications of decisions made during all phases of an emergency response. When it comes to public health emergencies, the effects can be more devastating to the medically fragile, especially when healthcare infrastructure fails. In these cases, all levels of government need to plan for health services and support the needs of the population in distress. Remember that major emergencies or disasters involving human casualties can severely challenge the ability of healthcare facilities and systems to provide care. Mitigating these risks is important to successful incident management.[4] We talk more about incident management within healthcare facilities in Chapter 13.

▶ Multiagency Coordination Systems (MACSs)

"As an incident becomes more complex, multiagency coordination becomes increasingly important. Multiagency coordination is a process that allows all levels of government and all disciplines to work together more efficiently and effectively."[5] The response is often hampered by conflicting policies, communication, and "turf" issues. To address these challenges, MACSs can be used to manage these more complex incidents that require greater interagency coordination. Effective multiagency coordination is defined by the system's ability to "provide reliable systems and resources to support the Incident Command; acquire, analyze and act on information; be flexible in the face of rapidly changing conditions; anticipate change; and promote public confidence."[5] The process is accomplished through a comprehensive system of elements: facilities, equipment, personnel, procedures, and communications.

It is important to understand that an MACS is not a physical location or facility, but rather a process. "A MAC system defines business practices, standard operating procedures and protocols by which participating agencies will coordinate their interactions. It provides support, coordination, and assistance with policy-level decisions to the ICS structure managing an incident. In addition, it helps define how cooperating agencies and organizations will work together more efficiently. MACS provide critical resource and information analysis support to the Incident Command/Unified Command. The primary functions of MACS include:

- Situation assessment
- Incident priority determination
- Critical resource acquisition and allocation
- Interagency activities"[5]

MACS generally perform common functions during an incident; however, not all of the system's functions will be performed during every incident, and functions may not occur in any particular order. MACSs may consist of several common coordination elements: dispatch center, emergency operations center (EOC), department operations center (DOC), and multiagency coordination (MAC) group[5]. See **FIGURE 9-2**.

"The Dispatch Center coordinates the acquisition, mobilization and movement of resources as ordered by the Incident Command/Unified Command. The Department Operations Center (DOC) coordinates an internal agency incident management and response. The EOC and MAC groups have a coordination and communication role in the process rather than command authority over the incident operations (**FIGURE 9-3** displays the communication role within MACSs). The Emergency Operations Center (EOC) supports the on-scene response by relieving the burden of external coordination and securing additional resources. Finally, the MAC group represents the agencies through their administrators and executives, or their designees, who are authorized to commit agency resources and funds."[5] There is no single policy for activating MACS elements. But MACSs can be activated when one or more jurisdictions becomes involved in the incident response or when the chief executive (e.g., mayor, governor, agency administrator, etc.) requests that MACS elements be activated.

It is critical to maintain the readiness of the MACS. After an incident, there are five steps that should be taken to prepare for the next incident:

1. Replenish resources
2. Update rosters, media lists and other contact information
3. Conduct tests, training and exercises
4. Maintain/update equipment
5. Follow up and implement recommendations from exercises[5]

The jurisdiction's emergency operations plan should identify who is responsible for carrying out these five steps.

How the system works

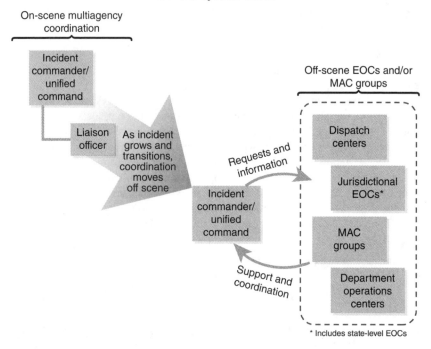

FIGURE 9-2 How the system works

Data from Federal Emergency Management Agency, Emergency Management Institute. IS-701a. NIMS Multiagency Coordination Systems Training Course. Available at: www.training.fema.gov/is/coursematerials.aspx?code=is-701.a. Accessed June 18, 2016.

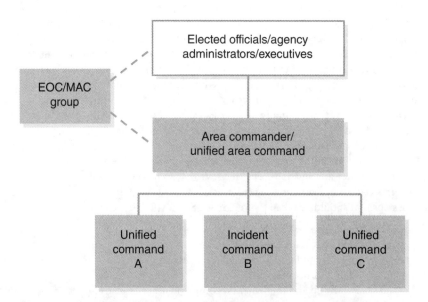

FIGURE 9-3 MACS's coordination and communication role

Data from Federal Emergency Management Agency, Emergency Management Institute. IS-701a. NIMS Multiagency Coordination Systems Training Course. Available at: www.training.fema.gov/is/coursematerials.aspx?code=is-701.a. Accessed June 18, 2016.

▶ Situational Awareness

Incident management occurs in a highly complex and rapidly changing environment. As a result, maintaining situational awareness at all times is an important aspect of incident management. Situational awareness is the ability to process and understand information, and how that information, events, and actions will impact the emergency. In addition to maintaining situational awareness to know how to best refine the response effort, emergency responders also need to communicate situational awareness to decision makers and elected officials, and the public. However, messages to the public may need to be tailored to avoid the communication of sensitive information that could compromise the response effort.

"The four priorities of situational awareness are:

1. Providing the right information at the right time.
2. Improving and integrating national reporting.
3. Linking operations centers and tapping subject-matter experts.
4. Standardizing reporting."[6]

"Situational awareness must start at the incident scene,"[5] and information must be effectively communicated across jurisdictions (local, state, and federal) and sectors (public, private, and nonprofit). The accuracy and timeliness of information and sharing thereof are a priority of situational awareness. This enables all parties to develop a clear understanding of the conditions on the ground and to plan the necessary response. Without accurate information, the effectiveness of the response will be jeopardized. "Jurisdictions must integrate existing reporting systems to develop an information and knowledge management system that fulfills national information requirements. Situational awareness is greatly improved when experienced technical specialists [and subject matter experts] identify critical elements of information"[5] and when that information is distributed broadly across operation centers. "The reporting and documentation procedures, including situation and status reports, should be standardized to provide emergency management and response personnel with access to critical information. Situation reports should contain verified information and explicit details (who, what, where, when and how) related to the incident. Status reports, which may be contained in situation reports, relay specific information about resources."[5]

▶ Information Sharing

During an emergency response, it is important to share and disseminate information and intelligence among disciplines and agencies, across jurisdictions and sectors, and between the various levels of government—federal, state, local, tribal, and territorial. The goal for any responder, particularly in public health, is to get the right information to the right people at the right time.

"Information sharing is the ability to conduct multijurisdictional, multidisciplinary exchange of health-related information and situational awareness data among federal, state, local, tribal, and territorial levels of government, as well as the private sector."[7(p55)] Information sharing is important in both preparedness and response activities. In the preparedness phase, public health professionals should establish communication pathways (internal and external), acquire or

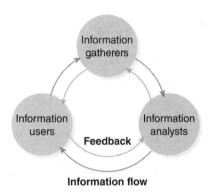

Information flow

FIGURE 9-4 Information flow

Data from Federal Emergency Management Agency, Emergency Management Institute. IS-701a. NIMS Multiagency Coordination Systems Training Course. Available at: www.training.fema.gov/is/coursematerials.aspx?code=is-701.a. Accessed June 18, 2016.

have access to redundant communication mechanisms, and identify partners with whom information needs to be shared. In the response phase, public health professionals need to ensure clear, consistent information flow to the public and response partners. An effective sharing and dissemination system provides reliable and effective information flow among information gatherers, analysts, and users, and allows for feedback among the information system participants, as illustrated in **FIGURE 9-4**.

As outlined in the Centers for Disease Control and Prevention's (CDC) Public Health Preparedness Capabilities, National Standards for State and Local Planning, Capability 6, information sharing should include the "routine sharing of information as well as issuing of public health alerts to federal, state, local, territorial, and tribal levels of government and the private sector in preparation for, and in response to, events or incidents of public health significance."[7(p55)]

▶ Communication and Information Systems

September 11, 2001, will forever be etched in the memories of many Americans as the deadliest attack on U.S. soil. Nearly 3000 people lost their lives, and many of those were first responders. Communications problems forced rescuers to make life-or-death decisions based on missing and/or incomplete information, and communications breakdowns also prevented evacuation announcements from reaching people inside the north tower before it fell.

Communications can be the difference between success and failure of any prevention or response effort, which is why effective and efficient communication is critical in all types of emergencies. Public officials must develop and implement measures that ensure effective communication with the public during emergencies and disasters. Inefficient communications, without safeguards to ensure transmission and reception of information, can weaken the disaster response. Information about the threat, as well as information about the response effort, is key to keeping the public informed and prepared to act. But communication does not merely start after an event. It is important to communicate with the public before the event to establish trust and develop relationships. Trust goes a long way in helping communities develop resilience.

The type of information that will need to be communicated, both within and outside response organizations, includes:

- Information about the threat
- What we know
- What we are doing
- What we do not know

During any emergency response, there will be multiple stakeholders, so both internal and external communications must be planned. Internally, among staff, topics such as work assignments, information sharing, status reporting, and call-down notifications regarding the situations will need to be addressed. Externally, you will have disparate audiences, including other responders (health departments, hospitals, community providers, ambulatory care providers, community partners, and volunteers), the general public (directly or indirectly affected by the emergency), and the media, which can help or harm the response. Each relevant audience should be addressed individually. For more on communicating with the public and media, see Chapter 11.

▶ Common Operating Picture

During an incident, a response involves the coordination of multiple agencies and many people from multiple disciplines working together. Developing a common understanding or common operating picture (COP) of the incident will enable the IC/Unified Command, supporting agencies, organizations, and individuals to make effective, consistent, and timely decisions. A COP is a shared situational awareness that offers a standard overview of an incident and provides information in a manner that enables incident leadership and any supporting agencies and organizations to make effective, consistent, coordinated, and timely decisions.[8(p21)] A COP will develop and maintain awareness across jurisdictions and organizations, ensuring consistency at all levels of incident management across and between sectors.

▶ Interoperable Communication

On September 11, 2001, after the planes had crashed into the World Trade Center, police officials had concluded the Twin Towers were in danger of collapsing and ordered police to leave the complex. Radio communications saved hundreds of police officers who received word to evacuate the building. Tragically, hundreds of New York firefighters did not receive the warning because they were using a different radio communications system, one that was not compatible, or interoperable, with the system used by the New York Police Department (NYPD).[9] In the federal 9/11 Commission Report and in appearances on news programs, city commissioners said the capabilities of communications systems lacked the ability to communicate across department lines. Police units could not communicate with fire units directly by radio. This ultimately impeded the coordination of the response effort and had enormous consequences to many of the responders. Ultimately, 343 fire-fighters lost their lives.[10]

As evidenced in the 9/11 response, interoperable communication systems are integral to any emergency response, not only for the ease of information sharing, but also to ensure that all responders obtain the same information related to the response effort. Interoperable communication refers to the "ability of emergency responders to communicate and share information and data, allowing emergency response personnel to communicate within their organizations and across other agencies and jurisdictions via voice, data or video."[11] Interoperable communication also includes the equipment needed to communicate, such as radio systems. If responders have physical communications systems that can directly communicate, those systems are considered to be interoperable. To be effective, interoperable communication must be compatible among multiple partners.[11] It requires integrated systems, interagency planning, and similar policies and processes across agencies. Furthermore, planners should build in redundancy in case of failure of the primary communication system or network.

▶ Information Sharing Agreements

In the midst of an emergency response, each participating agency and neighboring jurisdictions may have access to data that would help other participants to fulfill their missions and make the disaster response effort more efficient and effective. At the interagency level, medical records may be necessary to determine how to best treat patients. At the interjurisdictional level, one state may collect sentinel data on infectious diseases that would be useful for a neighboring state. But information sharing is typically constrained by technical, organizational, and political barriers.[12]

If a response is to be optimal, public health agencies and jurisdictions must be able to share certain data. For this reason, they may enter into an agreement to share specific public health or other emergency response data for a narrowly defined purpose. One example is the Great Lakes Border Health Initiative, a joint working group of eight partners who agreed to share "individually identifiable and population-related data for the purposes of preventing, detecting or responding to a public health event."[13(p. 2)] State laws vary in terms of permissible data sharing and requirements for data protection, and agencies should ensure they have thoroughly addressed potential legal issues.[14]

▶ Communication Systems and Communications Redundancy

The quality of communications systems can mean the difference between life and death. So, it is important to understand the various types of communication systems commonly in use. In public health, two communications systems that are frequently used in emergency response are the Epidemic Information Exchange (Epi-X) and Health Alert Network (HAN). Developed by the CDC, Epi-X is a secure, web-based communications network that allows for the exchange of information between CDC, state and local health departments, poison control centers, and other public health professionals. It also provides important disease information through surveillance alerts throughout the day. Epi-X will report outbreaks and alert health officials of urgent health events. It provides rapid reporting and instant notification, and assists in the coordination of health investigations for public health professionals.[15]

Also from the CDC, the HAN is a content-based emergency communication system that ensures communication capacity at local and state health departments by providing a forum for clinicians. HAN is the CDC's primary method for sharing information about urgent incidents with public information officers; federal, state, territorial, and local public health practitioners; clinicians; and public health laboratories. "HAN is a collaborative effort between federal, state, territorial, and city/county partners to develop protocols and help build stakeholder relationships that will ensure a robust interoperable platform for the rapid distribution of public health information."[16]

▶ Public Health Information Network (PHIN)

"Many organizations work together to protect and advance the public's health. These organizations operate a wide variety of public health information systems and need to reliably exchange critical and sensitive data among their disparate systems. Rather than attempting to integrate the various systems,"[17] the PHIN Messaging System (PHIN MS) is software that fulfills this critical need for public health. The PHIN is a national initiative to increase the capacity of public health agencies to electronically exchange data and information across organizations and jurisdictions. Established by the CDC, PHIN is designed to enhance early detection of public health emergencies and facilitate gathering, storage and dissemination of electronic information.[17]

▶ Syndromic Surveillance Systems

Syndromic surveillance systems are tools used in the analysis of medical data to detect or anticipate emerging disease outbreaks, and they can also be used to communicate information during emergency response. According to a CDC definition, "the term 'syndromic surveillance' applies to surveillance using health-related data that precede diagnosis and signal a sufficient probability of a case or an outbreak to warrant further public health response."[18] These systems collect data at the point of medical care and from existing data streams that can monitor and communicate disease patterns. Syndromic surveillance systems can also be useful in the detection of outbreaks attributable to bioterrorism.

The most effective syndromic surveillance systems automatically monitor existing systems in real time. They do not require individuals to enter separate information. The systems aggregate data from multiple systems using advanced analytical tools and provide automated alerts. For example, syndromic surveillance systems will monitor data from Internet searches, emergency call centers, emergency call systems, and other data sources to detect unusual patterns. When a significant change in activity is seen in any of the monitored systems, public health professionals or other relevant stakeholders are alerted that there may be an issue. This type of early warning system can limit the damage and number of casualties affected by an outbreak or bioterrorist attack.[18]

In 2008, Google launched Google Flu Trends to monitor flu-related searches that have been shown to correlate with higher flu activity and closely match CDC data that the Google system leads by 1–2 weeks.[19] But, like with any other model, there are limitations, and it should not be used in isolation or without expert supervision.[20] Syndromic surveillance systems have advantages and limitations. Although they do improve collaboration among stakeholders—healthcare providers, investigators, and public health agencies—they are not a substitute for direct physician reporting.

Two additional examples of syndromic surveillance systems are the Electronic Surveillance System for the Early Notification of Community-based Epidemics (ESSENCE) and the Real-time Outbreak and Disease Surveillance (RODS) system. ESSENCE monitors and delivers alerts for rapid or unusual increases in the occurrence of infectious diseases and biological outbreaks. It provides interactive reporting, structured analysis, ad hoc queries of disease syndromes, disease and injury categories, and reportable medical events.[21] Developed by the University of Pittsburgh's Department of Biomedical Informatics, RODS is free software for public health surveillance that collects and analyzes disease surveillance data from emergency departments within a geographic region in real time to provide a picture and early detection of epidemic events.[22]

▶ Conclusion

The importance of coordination and communication cannot be stressed enough when it comes to planning for an emergency response to a catastrophic event. While some emergencies will be small, localized, or require only one responding agency, larger, more complex emergencies will require response by multiple organizations. When this occurs, all responding organizations and disciplines need to operate within a defined system that is designed to foster coordination and effective communication throughout the response. An MAC System offers this process. MACSs support effective coordination among agency decision makers through the ICS by helping to define how cooperating agencies and organizations will work together efficiently throughout the response effort.

Emergency communications is a shared mission across all levels of government and sectors, and even with the public. Communication is the cornerstone for coordinating complex missions. During an emergency, public health professionals and other emergency responders must communicate with many audiences, with a different goal in each case.

It is important for responders to be able to provide and maintain communications before, during, and after an emergency. Inefficient communications without safeguards to ensure transmission and reception of information can weaken the disaster response. Disseminating information quickly, coordinating messages in a timely manner, and utilizing that information to ensure timely decision-making can minimize the damage and destruction of the disaster or emergency.

Discussion Questions

1. What is an MACS? How is it used in emergency response?
2. What are the primary functions of MACSs? Explain how MACSs help coordinate large, complex emergency response efforts.

3. What is the purpose of situational awareness during and after an emergency?
4. What is a COP? What is the goal of obtaining a COP?
5. Explain the benefit of an information sharing agreement.
6. In addition to the HAN, name three other communication systems, and briefly describe their purposes.
7. Explain how surveillance systems such as ESSENCE and RODS aid in emergency response communications. What in your opinion might be barriers to successful implementation of these systems?

References

1. U.S. Department of Homeland Security. NIMS: frequently asked questions. Available at https://www.fema.gov/pdf/emergency/nims/nimsfaqs.pdf. Accessed June 18, 2016.
2. U.S. Department of Homeland Security. Homeland security presidential directive 5. Available at https://www.dhs.gov/publication/homeland-security-presidential-directive-5. Accessed June 18, 2016.
3. Federal Emergency Management Agency, Emergency Management Institute. ICS Resource Center, ICS review document. Available at https://training.fema.gov/emiweb/is/icsresource/. Accessed June 18, 2016.
4. U.S. Department of Health and Human Services. *Medical Surge Capacity and Capability Handbook*. Available at https://www.phe.gov/Preparedness/planning/mscc/handbook/Documents/mscc080626.pdf. Published September 2007. Accessed June 18, 2016.
5. Federal Emergency Management Agency, Emergency Management Institute. IS-701a. NIMS Multiagency Coordination Systems Training Course. Available at https://training.fema.gov/is/coursematerials.aspx?code=is-701.a. Accessed June 18, 2016.
6. Federal Emergency Management Agency. Emergency Management Institute. IS-800b. National response framework training. Available at https://emilms.fema.gov/IS800B/lesson3/NRF0103180t.htm. Accessed June 18, 2016.
7. U.S. Centers for Disease Control and Prevention. Public health preparedness capabilities: national standards for state and local planning. Available at https://www.cdc.gov/phpr/readiness/00_docs/DSLR_capabilities_July.pdf. Published March 2011. Accessed July 26, 2016.
8. Federal Emergency Management Agency. National incident support manual. Available at https://www.fema.gov/media-library-data/20130726-1821-25045-8641/fema_national_incident_support_manual_03_23_2011.pdf. Published February 2011. Accessed March 18, 2017.
9. Dwyer J, Flynn K, Fessenden F. Fatal confusion: A troubled emergency response; 9/11 exposed deadly flaws in rescue plan. *New York Times*. Available at http://www.nytimes.com/2002/07/07/nyregion/fatal-confusion-troubled-emergency-response-9-11-exposed-deadly-flaws-rescue.html?mcubz=0. Published July 7, 2002. Accessed March 18, 2017.
10. National Commission on Terrorist Attacks upon the United States. 9/11 Commission Report. Available at https://9-11commission.gov/report/. Published July 22, 2004. Accessed March 18, 2017.
11. Disaster Resource Guide. Interoperable communication. Available at http://www.disaster-resource.com/index.php?option=com_content&view=article&id=859&Itemid=50. Accessed September 3, 2017.
12. Dawes SS. Interagency information sharing: Expected benefits, manageable risks. *J Policy Anal Manage*. 1996;15(3):377–394.
13. Great Lakes Border Health Initiative. Public health data sharing agreement. Available at https://www.michigan.gov/documents/mdch/2007-06-21_-_DATA_SHARING_AGREEMENT_202933_7.pdf. Updated February 2009. Accessed August 18, 2017.
14. Association of State and Territorial Health Officials. Public health information sharing toolkit. Public health and information sharing key issues and concepts. Available at http://www.astho.org/Programs/Preparedness/Public-Health-Emergency-Law/Public-Health-and-Information-Sharing-Toolkit/Key-Issues-and-Concepts-Overview/. Published 2012. Accessed August 18, 2017.

15. U.S. Centers for Disease Control and Prevention. Epidemic Information Exchange (Epi-X). Available at https://emergency.cdc.gov/epix/index.asp. Updated July 24, 2017. Accessed August 18, 2017.

16. U.S. Centers for Disease Control and Prevention. Health Alert Network (HAN). Available at https://emergency.cdc.gov/han/index.asp. Accessed August 18, 2017.

17. U.S. Centers for Disease Control and Prevention. PHIN tools and resources. Available at https://www.cdc.gov/phin/. Updated September 10, 2015. Accessed August 18, 2017.

18. Berger M, Shiau R, Weintraub JM. Review of syndromic surveillance: Implications for waterborne disease detection. *J Epidemiol Commun Health*. 2006;60(6):543–550. doi:10.1136/jech.2005.038539.

19. Ginsberg J, Mohebbi MH, Patel RS, Brammer L. Detecting influenza epidemics using search engine query data. *Nature*. 2009;457:1012–1014.

20. Salzberg S. Why Google is a Flu Failure. *Forbes Magazine*. Available at https://www.forbes.com/sites/stevensalzberg/2014/03/23/why-google-flu-is-a-failure/#7e3520355535. Published March 23, 2014. Accessed August 18, 2017.

21. Military Health System and the Defense Health Agency. Electronic surveillance system for the early notification of community-based epidemics. Available at https://health.mil/Military-Health-Topics/Technology/Clinical-Support/Centralized-Credentials-Quality-Assurance-System/Decision-Support/Electronic-Surveillance-System-for-the-Early-Notification-of-Community-based-Epidemics. Accessed August 18, 2017.

22. University of Pittsburgh. RODS laboratory. Available at http://www.rods.pitt.edu/site/content/view/15/36/. Accessed August 18, 2017.

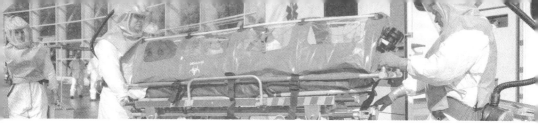

CHAPTER 10

Community Preparedness and Recovery

LEARNING OBJECTIVES

In all activities related to emergency preparedness, there is one driving goal: to help communities better prepare for, and recover from, disasters. Hazards and adverse events are inevitable in any society, and the job of public health professionals is to help ensure that people in all communities can withstand and manage through the shocks, stresses, and trauma of these incidents to ultimately emerge stronger than before. This chapter examines the role of public health in helping communities prepare and recover as quickly and effectively as possible. By the end of this chapter, readers should be able to:

- Understand the public health role in community preparedness
- Understand the public health role in community recovery
- Define psychological first aid
- Identify specific at-risk populations who may need additional support following an emergency or disaster
- Determine strategies for reaching and planning for at-risk populations

▶ Community Preparedness

As defined by the U.S. Centers for Disease Control and Prevention (CDC), community preparedness is the "ability of communities to prepare for, withstand, and recover—in both the short and long terms—from public health incidents."[1(pg.10)] For public health's responsibility in building and sustaining effective community preparedness capability, public health preparedness officials must engage and coordinate with multiple community stakeholders, both governmental and nongovernmental. Aside from planning with other emergency response partners, as discussed in previous chapters, public health emergency planners must undertake a variety of collaborative initiatives that include:

- Working with mental and behavioral health providers to make plans for addressing the psychosocial and psychological impacts of the disaster on the public and provide awareness training to community members.

- Leveraging relationships with community-based and faith-based partners on how to respond to public health incidents. Explore the possibility of training staff of these organizations so they can, in turn, provide training for more individuals in a "train-the-trainer" model. Community- and faith-based partners can also be instrumental in ensuring that public health messages, particularly risk communication messages, penetrate deep into the community and reach those whom government officials find most difficult to access and support.
- Engaging with public and private organizations that represent the unique cultural, socioeconomic, and demographic characteristics of the community.
- Engaging with organizations that serve at-risk, and vulnerable populations to help raise awareness, provide training, and plan for how to disseminate information, support, and resources to those communities in the event of a disaster.

The CDC Community Preparedness Capability also cites the following functions as part of public health's role in community preparedness:[1(p16)]

- Function 1: Determine risks to the health of the jurisdiction
- Function 2: Build community partnerships to support health preparedness
- Function 3: Engage with community organizations to foster public health, medical, and mental/behavioral health social networks
- Function 4: Coordinate training or guidance to ensure community engagement in preparedness efforts

In Chapter 7, we discussed community risk assessments and the importance of identifying potential hazards, risks, and vulnerabilities that exist within communities. In that context, risk assessment was critical as the first phase of the preparedness cycle, a preamble to the planning phase. In the context of community preparedness, risk assessments ensure that public health officials are aware of the full spectrum of risks to the jurisdiction's health and can plan for the provision of services—public health, medical, mental/behavioral health—in the event of occurrence of those risks. Armed with knowledge and understanding of the potential risks, public health is then able to determine what the needs of the community will be and can appropriately engage with partners to support preparedness efforts.

▶ Community Recovery

Community recovery refers to the ability to collaborate with community partners to plan and advocate for the rebuilding of systems to a level of function at least on par with, or better than, predisaster function. These systems can include health systems (medical, mental, and behavioral), transportation systems, government services, social services, education systems, and others.[1] In short, resilience and recovery are about how well a community can bounce back from the consequences of the emergency or disaster event, as close to pre-event functioning as possible.

The following functions are cited in CDC's Community Recovery Capability as functions that are integral to the role of public health in community recovery:[1(p22)]

- Function 1: Identify and monitor public health, medical, and mental/behavioral health system recovery needs

- Function 2: Coordinate community public health, medical, and mental/behavioral health system recovery operations
- Function 3: Implement corrective actions to mitigate damages from future incidents

It is important to understand that while public health officials have distinct roles in community recovery, there will never be a time when public health is performing any of their defined roles alone. In other words, all of the public health functions associated with community recovery will be carried out in the larger context of a community recovery effort, while working alongside other health and emergency management partners, as well as community partners.

Involvement by community partners in both preparedness and recovery cannot be overemphasized. No one knows the unique intricacies and complexities of specific communities better than those who live there. Community partners can assist preparedness officials in gaining a greater understanding of the needs of the community, which will inform and enhance preparedness plans. Additionally, as we have seen in recent history, some disasters will reveal characteristics about the community or new priorities for the community that must be embraced in order to build resilience for future disasters. This means some communities may need to change in order to build future resilience. It will be important for preparedness officials to have the input and support of community members in these situations, as it will make any necessary changes more acceptable to the community members who will be left to deal with them once recovery efforts have ended.[2]

In our post–Hurricane Katrina America, the importance of community preparedness and recovery ring loud daily. Whether due to climate change or other factors, the disasters that we see are becoming increasingly larger in scope and scale. Natural disasters of catastrophic proportions are occurring more frequently and consistently require response operations of epic magnitudes to protect communities and their greatest assets, citizens, property, and infrastructure systems. The massive devastation in New Orleans, Louisiana, and Joplin, Missouri, after Hurricane Katrina and the Joplin tornado on May 2011, respectively, demonstrates the importance of widespread community and stakeholder engagement in preparedness planning and response.

▶ Psychosocial Impacts of Disasters

Disaster events impact communities and individuals in different ways. Some of these impacts can be positive. For example, in the wake of disasters, communities may see a surge in volunteering, optimism, altruism, and social connectedness as people band together to help through donations of time, money, and needed supplies. But unsurprisingly, the psychological impacts of disasters are often negative and, for some individuals, can be long-lasting without professional assistance. Resilience is not only about the return of systems to normal levels of functioning; it is also about the return of individuals to normal levels of functioning. That is why a critically important responsibility of public health professionals is to ensure that individuals and the collective community have the resources necessary to return to a state of mental, behavioral, and physical health.

Even for people without diagnosed mental illness or other mental health concerns, the occurrence of an emergency or disaster can trigger significant mental health episodes such as anxiety, depression, and emotional instability. Other effects post-disaster can include physiological symptoms such as fatigue, gastrointestinal complaints, muscle tension, and increased heart rate; cognitive symptoms such as confusion, disorientation, and inability to concentrate; and behavioral changes such as insomnia, excessive sleeping, loss of appetite, withdrawal from others, and substance abuse.[3] For most affected people, these are temporary changes that they will be able to work through without professional help. For others, public health professionals must plan to have readily available resources to help individuals return to normal functioning and health. All planning activities should take these effects of disaster into account.

▶ Psychological First Aid

After any disaster, affected people may be confused, fearful, or angry. While these reactions are all normal, one in four survivors could develop long-term mental health issues such as depression or post-traumatic stress disorder (PTSD).[4] Psychological first aid (PFA) is an evidence-based approach designed to bolster the resilience of adults, children, adolescents, and families in the wake of a disaster. The main goal of PFA is to reduce stress symptoms and assist in a healthy recovery and avoid the potential for long-term psychological effects. PFA is not to be confused with traditional mental health or psychiatric treatment. Rather, it is simply a way to provide additional support and comfort that will lead to a sense of safety, calmness, connectedness, self-empowerment, and hope.

In 2012, the Chicago Department of Public Health (CDPH) developed training tools for residents and emergency officials to highlight the basics of psychological first aid. In the training materials, CDPH highlights the following PFA actions that can be implemented by professionals and laypersons to assist and comfort those experiencing high levels of stress following a traumatic event:

- Connecting with survivors and engaging in conversation
- Listening to their concerns, needs, and worries
- Acknowledging that their reactions are normal and common
- Helping people connect with friends, family, and community
- Helping people meet their physical needs, such as shelter, medication, and food
- Offering credible information and suggestions on services that can help

These approaches may be modified for children to make them developmentally and age appropriate. However, regardless of a survivor's age, PFA should never include telling people to "calm down" or advising them that "everything will be okay."[4] This could result in survivors feeling misunderstood and experiencing increased feelings of isolation. Finally, it is important to recognize that psychological damage that occurs in response to an event may not always be immediately evident. Emergency planners and preparedness officials should plan for the accommodation of mental/behavioral health services of varying degrees. Psychological first aid can help meet immediate needs until access to a mental health professional or other services is available.

Critical Incident Stress Management (CISM)

Although much of the focus of PFA is on those directly affected by a disaster, it is important that public health professionals include first responders in their plans as well. Throughout the course of a disaster response, police, firefighters, military personnel, and health workers may be exposed to situations that are unsettling, at best, and severely traumatizing, at worst. First responders' efforts in emergencies can make them susceptible to the development or exacerbation of mental health conditions.[5] Because a community's ability to recover depends directly on the effectiveness of first responders and front-line workers, it is critically important to ensure their mental health.

Critical Incident Stress Management (CISM) is a short-term program that works to decrease stress in the early stages of a disaster and post-disaster to prevent stress reactions from taking root.[6] CISM was designed for first responders and may include preincident preparedness, crisis management, and postcrisis follow-up. It comprises seven steps[7]:

1. Precrisis preparation, including stress management education, stress resistance, and crisis mitigation training for both individuals and organizations
2. Disaster or large-scale incident, as well as school and community support programs including demobilizations, informational briefings, town meetings, and staff advisement
3. Defusing, which is a three-phase, structured small-group discussion provided within hours of a crisis for purposes of assessment, triaging, and acute symptom mitigation
4. Critical Incident Stress Debriefing (CISD), which is a seven-step structured group discussion, usually provided 1–10 days postcrisis and is designed to mitigate acute symptoms, assess the need for follow-up, and, if possible, provide a sense of postcrisis psychological closure
5. One-on-one crisis intervention/counseling or psychological support throughout the full range of the crisis spectrum
6. Family crisis intervention as well as organizational consultation
7. Follow-up and referral mechanisms for assessment and treatment, if necessary

Debriefing/Crisis Counseling

Debriefing, which is Step 4 of the CISM model, is a specific technique designed to assist individuals and groups in dealing with any psychological symptoms after trauma exposure. The goal of a debriefing is to provide a safe, confidential space in which those involved with the incident—whether as first responders or community members—can process the event and reflect on its impact, gradually working through the psychological trauma. Debriefing may also be helpful in reentry back into normal functioning in the community or workplace.

Debriefing should focus on the following points:[8]

1. Auditing/assessing impacts of the incident on support personnel and survivors
2. Identifying immediate issues surrounding problems related to safety and security

3. Defusing to allow people to vents their thoughts, emotions, and experiences associated with the event; providing validation of reactions
4. Predicting events and reactions to come in an event's aftermath
5. Conducting a systematic review of the critical incident and its emotional, physical, and cognitive impact; watching for maladaptive behaviors or responses to the trauma or crisis
6. Bringing closure to the incident and, if possible, helping participants to identify positive experiences from the event

Family Assistance Centers

Often, in the wake of an incident, local communities will partner with the Red Cross to establish Family Assistance Centers (FACs). The Family Assistance Center (FAC) model is a "framework for providing family assistance" following an emergency or disaster.[9(pg.2)] This concept is based on the need to provide families with a safe location where information exchange can take place following disasters, family members have privacy to process or grieve the effects of the disaster, and staff can facilitate the provision of emergency support services. Historically, these centers were designed for implementation following mass casualty events, such as terrorism events or aviation emergencies,[9] but over time their usage has expanded to other types of large-scale events as well. FACs provide private spaces where victims and their family members can meet with professional staff from multiple agencies and disciplines who can assist with the recovery process following a disaster. These professionals can include disaster mental health workers, health services personnel, and case workers who can assess the emergency needs of individuals and communities.[10] FACs also provide for basic needs such as meals, snacks, and water. For children, these centers can include specialists in children's mental health and therapeutic play. In some cases, FACs may even be able to connect individuals with financial assistance in the aftermath of a disaster.

▶ At-Risk Populations

Define At-Risk Populations

It is difficult to overstate the importance of addressing at-risk populations (also called vulnerable, special, or functional needs populations) in all planning and response at the federal, state, tribal, territorial, and local levels. These populations include persons who have specific life circumstances that may make it harder for them than others to access public health, medical, or other services they may require after a disaster or emergency. They also may need additional assistance in the areas of communication, medical care, supervision, or transportation. Some examples of at-risk populations include:

- Children
- Senior citizens
- Those with limited English proficiency
- Hearing and visually impaired
- Physically disabled

- Mentally impaired
- Those with low socioeconomic status
- Pregnant women
- Those who are homebound
- Institutionalized individuals (nursing homes, jails)
- Chronically ill
- Transportation disadvantaged
- Pharmacologically dependent

Because additional support and resources may be needed for these groups, planners and officials must ensure that emergency plans consider the needs of at-risk populations. Locating at-risk populations and planning for their needs can help ensure a more successful response to their specific situations during a disaster.

Locating At-Risk Populations

To identify at-risk individuals, public health workers and emergency planners should engage and partner with organizations that routinely service and provide care to them. Government agencies can be useful sources to identify these organizations, as can faith-based organizations, universities, and ethnic groups. Digital mapping software can also assist public health planners in identifying the locations of at-risk populations.

Regardless of how these groups are located, it is important to know that they must be regularly engaged to ensure awareness remains a priority. As is often said among many at-risk communities, "nothing for us without us." These communities know their needs best and want to be involved in the planning process. At-risk communities can themselves be a valuable asset to emergency planners as the planners explore different resources that could be used to meet the range of needs in the particular community following a disaster.

Reaching At-Risk Populations

Because at-risk populations become more vulnerable during disasters, it is important that plans include effective communication modalities to reach these population groups. Public health workers must be able to identify the best communication methods to use to share emergency information with at-risk groups before, during, and after disasters. In an emergency, messages must inform, educate, and mobilize people to follow public health directives. "Messages can be delivered through television, radio, newspaper, social media, bill inserts, flyers, word-of-mouth, social and community networks, and other channels"[11]. In an effort to assist emergency planners with identifying at-risk populations, the National Center for Environmental Health (NCEH) at the CDC created guidance that includes processes and tools that can help in identifying these groups. Information contained in the guidance document is designed to assist emergency planners in reducing vulnerabilities and improving outcomes for at-risk populations following a disaster.[11]

As indicated in the guide, community-based response efforts can be designed and implemented during all phases of a disaster. **TABLE 10-1** is a depiction of specific efforts that can be implemented and the appropriate times to do so.

TABLE 10-1 Use of Information for At-Risk Groups	
Phase	**Use of Information**
Preparedness	■ Create evacuation and contingency plan ■ Conduct community outreach and engagement ■ Determine resource needs and allocation ■ Prepare shelter, supplies, transportation, and evacuation plans
Response	■ Determine resource allocation ■ Provide targeted data to decision makers and first responders ■ Prioritize response efforts ■ Tailor communication efforts
Recovery	■ Determine resource allocation ■ Identify subpopulations that are the least resilient ■ Track recovery and identify ongoing problems
Mitigation	■ Develop hazard mitigation plans ■ Set up community shelters ■ Develop structural planning and policies

Data from CDC. Planning for an Emergency: Strategies for Identifying and Engaging At-Risk Groups. Available at: www.cdc.gov /nceh/hsb/disaster/atriskguidance.pdf. Accessed: August 18, 2017.

▶ Trusted Agents

The need to plan is particularly important in communities where communication with government agencies is either difficult or suspect, and where a more trusted figure could create a bridge between emergency responders and citizens. For example, in certain communities, government representatives may be distrusted. This lack of trust was a contributing factor in the decision of many New Orleans residents to ignore evacuation warnings during Hurricane Katrina in 2005, resulting in injuries, deaths, and emergency rescues.[12] In other communities, such as the visually or hearing impaired, physically disabled, or those who are not proficient in English, citizens may simply be unable to consume information in a traditional format and thus could be difficult to reach with emergency details and instructions in the midst of a disaster.

In these communities, public health departments must identify liaisons who are trusted by citizens and can serve as conduits of information. These leaders can provide valuable insight into the special resource needs and characteristics of a community to help agencies spread awareness and prepare for emergencies, as well as disseminate information during an incident. Examples of trusted community figures include faith-based leaders, leaders of local nonprofit organizations, representatives of clubs or affinity groups, advocacy groups, disability organizations, and other community partners.

▶ Conclusion

The goal of community preparedness and recovery is to develop the capability to assist communities to better prepare for and recover from disasters. Development of these capabilities can be dependent on a number of factors including engagement, partnership, advocacy, identification of the socially vulnerable, and trust. In planning to address the public health, medical, and mental/behavioral health needs of community residents following a disaster, these factors will all need to be considered by emergency planners and acted upon. There are tools available to assist emergency planners in developing these capabilities; however, those tools need to be identified and understood so they are able to be fully utilized during both the planning and response phases. Tools such as PFA and CISM aid in decreasing stress and mental health trauma among disaster victims after an event has occurred. FACs provide safe spaces for family members to relax, regroup, receive service, and debrief following disaster events. FACs can also create opportunities for emergency responders to obtain information or reconnect families with loved ones following an emergency. During the planning phase, tools such as geospatial information systems and policy guidance can assist planners in both locating at-risk populations and planning for their needs. However, the most important tool available to emergency planners in their community preparedness and recovery efforts are community members. As the persons who have the highest level of interest in the community post-disaster, community members can be valuable assets in capability development, including community members who are part of an at-risk or socially vulnerable group within the community. It is important for emergency planners to understand the full expanse of available tools to help achieve these capabilities.

Discussion Questions

1. Define community preparedness.
2. What is public health's role in community preparedness planning?
3. What is the primary goal of PFA?
4. What are two statements that should never be spoken to a victim when PFA is being implemented?
5. Name three at-risk populations groups. What are some challenges these groups might face during and after an emergency or disaster? How can emergency planners ensure planning efforts consider these challenges and mitigate them?

References

1. U.S. Centers for Disease Control and Prevention. Public health preparedness capabilities: national standards for state and local planning, March 2011. Available at https://www.cdc .gov/phpr/readiness/00_docs/DSLR_capabilities_July.pdf.
2. Gurwitch RH, Pfefferbaum B, Montgomery JM, Klomp RW, Reissman DB. *Building Community Resilience for Children and Families*. Oklahoma City: Terrorism and Disaster Center at the University of Oklahoma Health Sciences Center; 2007. Available at http://www.nctsnet.org /nctsn_assets/pdfs/edu_materials/BuildingCommunity_FINAL_02-12-07.pdf.

3. Psychological First Aid. National child traumatic stress network. Available at http://www .nctsn.org/content/psychological-first-aid. Accessed July 13, 2017.

4. Chicago Department of Public Health. Psychological first aid video. Available at https:// www.cityofchicago.org/city/en/depts/cdph/provdrs/health_protection/news/2012/sep/new _training_toolshighlightpsychologicalfirstaidbasics.html.

5. Benedek DM, Fullerton C, Ursano RJ. First responders: Mental health consequences of natural and human-made disasters for public health and public safety workers. *Annu Rev Public Health.* 2007;28:55–68.

6. Pulley SA, Critical Incident Stress Management. eMedicine from WedMD. Available at https:// web.archive.org/web/20060811232118/http:/www.emedicine.com/emerg/topic826.htm. Accessed July 13, 2017.

7. Everly GS, Mitchell JT. A primer on critical incident stress management. International Critical Incident Stress Foundation, Inc. Available at https://www.icisf.org/a-primer-on -critical-incident-stress-management-cism/. Accessed July 13, 2017.

8. Mitchell J, Everly GS. *Critical Incident Stress Debriefing: An Operations Manual for the Prevention of PTSD Among Emergency Services and Disaster Workers.* Ellicott City, MD: Chevron Publishing Corporation; 1996.

9. U.S. Department of Justice. Mass fatality incident family assistance operations, recommended strategies for local and state agencies. Available at https://ntsb.gov/tda/TDADocuments /Mass%20Fatality%20Incident%20Family%20Assistance%20Operations.pdf. Accessed August 18, 2017.

10. American Red Cross. Family Assistance Center in Boston helps families of victims heal. Available at http://www.redcross.org/news/article/Family-Assistance-Center-in-Boston-Helps -Families-of-Victims-Heal. Accessed August 18, 2017.

11. U.S. Centers for Disease Control and Prevention. Planning for an Emergency: strategies for identifying and engaging at-risk groups, 2015. Available at https://www.cdc.gov/nceh/hsb /disaster/atriskguidance.pdf. Accessed August 18, 2017.

12. Cordasco KM, Eisenman D, Glik DC, Golden JF, Asch SM. They blew the levee: distrust of authorities among Hurricane Katrina evacuees. *J Health Care Poor Underserved.* 2007;18(2): 277–282.

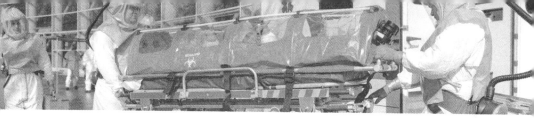

CHAPTER 11

Crisis and Emergency Risk Communication

▶ Emergency Public Information and Warning

As defined in the Centers for Disease Control and Prevention's (CDC) Public Health Preparedness Capabilities, emergency public information and warning is the ability to develop, coordinate, and disseminate information, warnings, and notifications to the public and to incident management responders. To fulfill this capability, organizations must have the ability to do the following:

- Function 1: Activate the emergency public information system
- Function 2: Determine the need for a joint public information system

- Function 3: Establish and participate in information system operations
- Function 4: Establish avenues for public interaction and information exchange
- Function 5: Issue public information alerts, warnings, and notifications[1]

▶ Public Information

"Public information consists of the processes, procedures, and systems for communicating timely, accurate, and accessible information on an incident's cause, size, and current situation; resources committed; and other matters of general interest to the public, responders, and additional stakeholders, both directly and indirectly affected. Public information, education strategies, and communications plans help ensure that numerous audiences receive timely, consistent messages about lifesaving measures, evacuation routes, threat and alert system notices, and other public safety information".[2] Within public health agencies, the staff role responsible for leading the development and dissemination of these messages is the public information officer (PIO). The PIO is responsible for carrying out public information functions, ensuring they are coordinated and integrated across jurisdictions and across functional agencies; among federal, state, local, and tribal partners; and with private-sector and nongovernmental organizations (NGOs).[2]

Public Information Officers

As with all communication strategies, the goal of a public information campaign should be to get the right information to the right people at the right time. PIOs should be skilled in message development and dissemination and should also be well-skilled at managing the media. The PIO is a key staff member within the

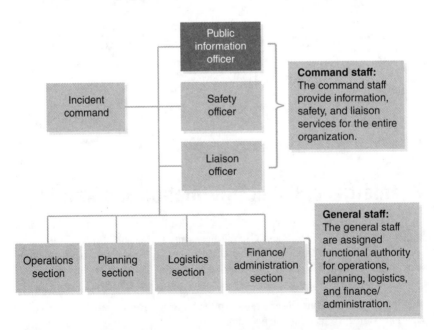

FIGURE 11-1 Role of the PIO

Data from Federal Emergency Management Agency. Emergency Management Institute. IS-702a. NIMS Public Information. Available at: www.emilms.fema.gov/IS702A/ Accessed: August 3, 2017.

incident command structure. In the Incident Command System (ICS), the PIO advises and represents the incident command on all public information matters relating to the management of the incident and may also serve as the spokesperson for the response. **FIGURE 11-1** displays the role of the PIO within the ICS.

Outside of the ICS structure, PIOs typically communicate directly with the media, which is why this role is often filled by someone with prior media industry experience. While the details will vary from one disaster to another, PIOs need to provide information to the public that is clear, concise, and informative. Typically, in emergency situations, members of the public are looking for information that will enable them to gain facts about the emergency, empower decision-making, and enable them to protect themselves and family members, as well as obtain information about the cause of the incident and what is being done to mitigate it.[3]

The PIO's answers to the public's questions matter tremendously in an emergency response, more than it might seem. Accurate responses have the potential to save lives. But inaccurate, misleading, or untimely answers not only may risk lives in the immediate aftermath, but also may sow long-lasting distrust in government, which will lead to worse outcomes in the future. A lack of trust in government representatives in times of crisis generally stems from the perception that promises have been broken or a community's values have been violated.[4]

To avoid these pitfalls in communication, PIOs must share information early, acknowledge the concerns of the public continuously, never be condescending in tone, and always deliver on promises. Key tactics for PIOs may include:

- Focusing on one or two key messages
- Using pre-scripted messages and talking points when appropriate
- Designating spokespeople for media interviews
- Speaking about their own programs, not about others' programs

PIOs will typically need to answer different types of questions from the media, who often want to understand the causes of and context surrounding the disaster. Members of the media will frequently place significant demands for information on PIOs. PIOs should recognize the media will demand rapid information, and will insist that information be provided constantly. It is a well-known fact that not all incident information will be available immediately. Therefore, PIOs should prepare to provide information to the media when it is available, and be sure to keep channels open with the media, so messages are both communicated and received in a timely manner.[3]

Joint Information Systems

When multiple agencies are involved in the response, PIOs from each agency will need to closely work together to coordinate public information messages. Message coordination is typically conducted via a Joint Information System (JIS). A JIS provides the mechanism to organize, integrate, and coordinate information to ensure timely, accurate, accessible, and consistent messaging across multiple jurisdictions and disciplines with NGOs and the private sector. The JIS includes the plans, protocols, procedures, and structures used to provide public information. In essence, a JIS is a way for multiple agencies to speak with one voice. As such, it provides clarity and prevents public confusion that would result from mixed messages emanating from different agencies. A JIS can take multiple forms of varying complexity:

- Two PIOs collaborating on the phone to address an incident that involves both of their agencies

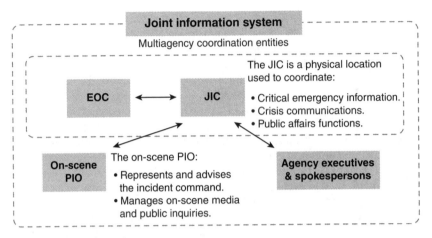

FIGURE 11-2 Role of the JIS

Data from Federal Emergency Management Agency. Emergency Management Institute. IS-702a. NIMS Public Information. Available at: www.emilms.fema.gov/IS702A/ Accessed: August 3, 2017.

- A PIO at the emergency operations center (EOC) talking to a PIO at the site of the incident
- PIOs from several departments working together at a single location
- Many PIOs from many agencies working together from several locations[2]

While a JIS ensures a consistent, unified voice in a time of crisis, it is important to understand that the agencies or departments that participate in the JIS do not lose their individual identities or responsibilities during a disaster. **FIGURE 11-2** displays the relationship between the PIO and the JIS.

Joint Information Centers

It is important to understand that the JIS is not a physical location but rather people, resources, and organizations working together in a coordinated manner. When this coordination is done in a physical facility or location, that location is called the Joint Information Center (JIC). The JIC is a central location in which the JIS operates. It is the place from where crisis communications and public affairs functions emanate. A JIC may be established at various levels of government or at incident sites, or can be a component of multiagency coordination systems (MACSs). While a single JIC location is ideal, the JIS should be flexible enough to accommodate multiple locations, including virtual locations, as circumstances may require.[3]

▶ Crisis and Emergency Risk Communication

Crisis and Emergency Risk Communication (CERC) is a CDC-developed training program based on the premise that "the right message at the right time from the right person can save lives."[3] It gives public health professionals in general, and PIOs specifically a framework for what to say, how to say it, and when to say it during an emergency. CERC combines crisis communication, which is related to emergency management of an unexpected and threatening incident, with risk communication, which is information about the expected outcome of a behavior or exposure. It gives individuals and communities enough information to make quick and sometimes extremely conse-quential decisions about their own well-being. Failure to apply the principles of CERC may result in a failure to communicate information that could save lives.

CERC is useful because it acknowledges that during crises, normal plans and procedures for communicating with the public may be inadequate. Crises by definition are full of uncertainty, and they cannot be adequately managed by simply adding more people to the emergency response. During crisis situations, decision makers are often unable to collect and process information in a timely manner, so they cannot rely on standard routines for situations that are anything but routine.[3]

"Communication during a crisis requires a different mindset. In major disas-ters, the incident may be so shattering that the basic understanding of what is occurring and the means to rebuild that understanding fall apart."[3] CERC provides a framework to deal with this level of uncertainty without compromising the impor-tance of timely public communication. The six principles of CERC are as follows:

1. **Be first.** Crises are time sensitive, and communicating information quickly is almost always important. For members of the public, the first source of information often becomes the preferred source.
2. **Be right.** Accuracy establishes credibility. Information can include what is known, what is not known, and what is being done to fill in the gaps.
3. **Be credible.** Honesty and truthfulness should not be compromised during crises.
4. **Express empathy.** Crises create harm, and the suffering should be acknowledged in words. Addressing what people are feeling, and the challenges they face, builds trust and rapport.
5. **Promote action.** Giving people meaningful things to do calms anxiety, helps restore order, and promotes a restored sense of control.
6. **Show respect.** Respectful communication is particularly important when people feel vulnerable. Respectful communication promotes cooperation and rapport.

Despite the chaotic nature of crises, public health communicators must be on guard for common pitfalls that can impede crisis communications, imperil a response, and compromise future trust of the public. Those failures include the following:[3,4]

- **Mixed messages from multiple experts.** Mixed messages convey the impres-sion that a response is uncoordinated and incompetent. Through the JIS, PIOs can ensure that a clear, unified message emerges from their own communica-tions and those funneled through the media.
- **Information released late or not at all.** If necessary, explain why the informa-tion is not available and when it will be available. It is important to not withhold information that will be useful to the public, even if that information is poten-tially embarrassing to a government agency.
- **Overly paternalistic attitudes.** People want information so they can make their own decisions about how to proceed. Paternalistic attitudes imply that the government knows what is best for a person even more than a person knows about themselves, which can come across as arrogance to someone who is feel-ing powerless and disenfranchised.
- **Not countering rumors and myths in real time.** Rumors and myths can build and travel at an alarming rate. Public health communicators must set the

record straight early and often, sometimes in partnership with trusted agents in at-risk communities.

- **Public power struggles and conflicts.** Power struggles between agencies will serve only to undermine an emergency response and the community's trust in the government's ability to assist in times of crisis. Emergency response plans should be thorough and clear enough that power struggles will not occur; if they do, they must remain out of the public eye and be resolved swiftly.
- **Spokespeople who exhibit a lack of appropriate emotion or use inappropriate humor.** Sincerity is critical in addressing individuals whose communities are in a state of disaster. Spokespeople must display the right mix of empathy and assurance.
- **Overpromising outcomes.** Instead, public health communicators should acknowledge the uncertainty of the situation as well as confidence that the process in place will fix the problem and address public safety concerns.

▶ Working with the Media

Disasters are not just major public health events. They are major media events, often generating wall-to-wall coverage in local and national media, sometimes for days. Working with the media in times of crisis can be stressful and time-consuming, particularly in cases when a disaster is ongoing or worsening. It is easy to slip into a mindset that views the media as a distraction during times of high stress and uncertainty, but in reality, the media is a critical partner during an incident. Without media, it would be difficult for agencies to disseminate their messages to the masses in a timely manner. That is why all public health communicators must develop positive working relationships with the media long before a disaster occurs. Some ways to nurture these relationships are to regularly communicate with media about preparedness and awareness campaigns and to invite local media to EOCs prior to an event so they can learn how information will be disseminated during an incident.

Some responsibilities of a PIO in working with the media include the following:

- Review common responsibilities
- Determine if there are limits on releasing information
- Develop material for use in media briefings
- Obtain approval for said briefings
- Inform media/conduct briefings
- Arrange for tours and briefings, as required
- Obtain media information that may be useful in incident planning
- Maintain current information summaries or displays on the incident
- Provide information on the status of the event to assigned personnel
- Maintain activity logs

Verification

In the midst of an incident, information may be difficult to control, particularly in the age of social media, where individuals with smartphones can circumvent traditional media and disseminate their own points of view, personal accounts of events, and even second- or third-hand accounts of events—some of which may be slanted, misleading, or inaccurate. Public health communicators have a special responsibility to verify information before allowing it to be released to the public. Before releasing information to the public, communicators must consider the source. Is the source credible? Is the characterization plausible? Is it consistent with other accounts?

Notification and Coordination

After verifying information to the best of one's abilities, public health communicators must notify managers in their own organization immediately, leaving out anything that has not been verified. Next, it is important to coordinate with other members of the organization and outside partners, if necessary. For example, if a public health professional is alerted to an incident by a reporter, the first step is to notify the director of the organization and only then to reach out to partner organizations that may be involved in a response.

Answering Questions

Members of the media will ask some of the same questions that members of the public want answered about the emergency. However, they frequently ask other questions that dig deeper into the context of a crisis, for example:

- Who is in charge?
- How are those who got hurt getting help?
- Is this event being contained?
- Why did this happen? (Do not speculate. Repeat the facts of the event, describe the data collection effort, and describe treatment from fact sheets.)
- Did you know ahead of time that this might happen?
- Why wasn't this kept from happening (again)?
- What else can go wrong?
- When did you begin working on this (were notified of this, determine this)?
- What do these data (information, results) mean?
- What bad things aren't you telling us?[3]

Ensuring Fairness

PIOs and other public health communicators will need to interact with multiple news organizations throughout a crisis period. It is important to provide equal access to all legitimate media outlets to promote a sense of fairness. Likewise, providing information to all media at once—whether through distribution lists, teleconferences, or on-site press conferences—will give reporters the sense that the government response is coordinated, fair, and responsive.

Local media, while smaller in reach and footprint, should never be overlooked in favor of larger national outlets. Local media typically has a keener understanding of local issues and communities and may be seen by the public as a more trusted source of local information.

▶ Other Mechanisms for Communicating

While the public may rely heavily on traditional media as a source of information during a crisis, public health communicators have many other avenues for disseminating critical information.

Emergency Alert System

The Emergency Alert System (EAS) is a national public warning system that requires broadcasters, cable TV systems, wireless cable systems, satellite digital audio radio services, and direct broadcast satellite services to provide the communications capability to the President to address the American public during a national emergency.[5] The EAS is maintained by the Federal Communications Commission (FCC), the Federal Emergency Management Agency (FEMA), and the National Weather Service (NWS). EAS may also be used by state and local authorities to deliver information about weather-related and other imminent threats.

Integrated Public Alert and Warning System

The Integrated Public Alert and Warning System (IPAWS) is a system that can send brief wireless emergency alerts that appear on mobile phones like text messages.[6]

Phone Banks

During localized emergency events, jurisdictions may establish phone banks as a mechanism for information dissemination to the public. Frequently used by public health agencies during large outbreaks, phone banks provide the general public with a mechanism for actively gathering information about the event from responding agencies. Phone banks are staffed by public health advisors, or epidemiologists, or other personnel with a working knowledge of the event and the ability to answer questions from the public.

Triage Lines

To effectively deal with a surge in patients that can happen during a disaster, healthcare providers may set up triage phone lines as a way to determine who needs treatment, advise any non-urgent cases on how to provide at-home treatment, and direct those in need of treatment to the best location for medical intervention. When members of the public call these triage lines, those who answer the phone can use the opportunity to provide other important information about what to do.

Social Media

While not an emergency communication system, social media is quickly becoming an alternative mechanism by which the general public obtains news and information. Facebook, Twitter, Instagram, and Snapchat, among other social networks, are now being used almost constantly and in very near real time to obtain and disseminate information. "Social media is expanding not only the scope and type of PIO work activity, but also the 'information pathways' that exist between PIOs, the media, and members of the public."[7] Social media is changing the way our society communicates; hence, emergency planners, communications officials, and PIOs should embrace and become comfortable with the use of social media in response efforts.[8]

▶ Communication Planning

A crisis communications plan is a critical document that requires extensive consideration, development, and review so that when a disaster happens, all participants in the communications aspect of a response effort will thoroughly understand their roles and responsibilities and feel equipped to carry them out according to the plan. All emergency response plans should contain communication annexes or sections, and communication plans should describe:

- How messages will be communicated
- What information is needed
- How information will be gathered quickly
- What the communication pathways are to other agencies
- How public information materials will be released

National Emergency Communication Plan

The Department of Homeland Security (DHS) Office of Emergency Communications (OEC) developed the National Emergency Communications Plan (NECP) to serve as the nation's first strategic plan for emergency communications guidance. It sets forth five goals and associated recommendations to enhance emergency communications capabilities at all levels of government and across disciplines in coordination with the private sector, NGOs, and communities:[9]

- **Governance and leadership:** Enhance decision-making, coordination, and planning for emergency communications through strong governance structures and leadership.
    - Update governance structures and processes to address the evolving operating environment.
    - Increase intrastate collaboration of communications, broadband, and information technology activities.
    - Increase regional structures or processes to foster multistate coordination and information sharing.
    - Enable the Emergency Communications Preparedness Center to serve as the federal focal point for coordination with the First Responder Network Authority.
    - Increase coordination of public safety and national security and emergency preparedness communications requirements and policies.
    - Promote opportunities to share federal emergency communications infrastructure and resources.
    - Promote consistent policies across federal grant programs and investments.
    - Improve the ability to assess the impact of emergency communications grant funding.
- **Planning and procedures:** Update plans and procedures to improve emergency responder communications and readiness in a dynamic operating environment.
    - Update Statewide Communications Interoperability Plans to maintain Land Mobile Radio systems and address wireless broadband deployments.
    - Coordinate federal strategic planning for broadband capabilities through the Emergency Communications Preparedness Center.

- Enable one DHS to lead the implementation of a DHS strategic plan for emergency communications.
- Ensure nationwide public safety broadband planning is coordinated throughout each state and territory and focuses on responders' current and future needs.
- Establish points of contact to coordinate federal broadband planning and deployment activities.
- Expand life-cycle planning activities to address broadband deployments and security, as needed.
- Evaluate, update, and distribute standard operating procedures to address new technologies and align them to tactical plans.
- Ensure standard operating procedures reflect current use of priority telecommunications services.
- Coordinate with entities from across the broader emergency response community to develop communications standard operating procedures.

- **Training and exercises:** Improve responders' ability to coordinate and communicate through training and exercise programs that use all available technologies and target gaps in emergency communications.
  - Develop training and exercise programs that target gaps in emergency communications capabilities and use new technologies.
  - Identify opportunities to integrate more private- and public-sector communications stakeholders into training and exercises.
  - Increase responder proficiency with federal and national interoperability channels through training and exercises.
  - Use regional governance structures to develop and promote training and exercise opportunities.
  - Leverage technologies, conferences, and workshops to increase training and exercise opportunities.
  - Promote awareness of and cross-training among federal, state, local, tribal, and territorial ICS Communications Unit personnel through training and exercises.
  - Develop and share best practices on processes to recognize trained Communications Unit personnel.
  - Improve states' and territories' ability to track and share trained Communications Unit personnel during response operations.

- **Operational coordination:** Ensure operational effectiveness through the coordination of communications capabilities, resources, and personnel from across the whole community.
  - Ensure inventories of emergency communication resources are updated and comprehensive.
  - Enhance jurisdictions' ability to readily request communications resources or assets during operations.
  - Implement ICS communications-related roles, responsibilities, and planning.
  - Ensure operational planning incorporates new technologies and communications partners.
  - Ensure Public Safety Answering Point and Public Safety Communications Center continuity of operations planning addresses systems and staffing to support dispatch communications.

- Update procedures for implementing backup communications solutions.
- Increase federal departments' and agencies' preparation and support for local emergency communications needs.

■ **Research and development:** Coordinate research, development, testing, and evaluation activities to develop innovative emergency communications capabilities that support the needs of emergency responders.

- Coordinate federal research and development priorities and user requirements through the Emergency Communications Preparedness Center.
- Increase collaboration between federal research and development and technology transfer programs across the homeland security, defense, and national security communities.
- Foster collaborative mission critical voice, data, and cybersecurity research, development, testing, and evaluation.
- Government research facilities should facilitate the integration of Next Generation 9-1-1 into a nationwide solution.
- Cultivate an innovative marketplace for applications and technologies through the use of public and private partnerships.
- Support the evolution of alert and warning systems that deliver timely, relevant, and accessible emergency information to the public.
- Update priority service programs to successfully migrate to Internet Protocol–enabled fixed and mobile broadband networks.
- Increase use and awareness of the Project 25 Compliance Assessment Program.
- Continue to support Project 25 standards development for interoperability.

▶ Cultural Competence and Cultural Humility

The diversity of the U.S. population is growing every year, and research has demonstrated that at-risk groups, such as minority populations, may be more susceptible to, and recover more slowly from, disasters, due in part to cultural barriers that public health officials may be ill-prepared to overcome.[10]

Public health professionals must be prepared to address the needs of many different racial, ethnic, and special populations, all within the context of a single emergency event. To develop that capability, they need cultural competence. Cultural competence refers to the ability of an organization to deliver services that meet the social, cultural, and linguistic needs of a particular community. Organizations must build cultural competency into disaster communications plans to ensure the fair and just treatment of at-risk populations before, during, and after a disaster. These populations can include races, ethnicities, sexual orientations, faiths, religions, and more.

The Department of Health and Human Services Office of Minority Health defines five elements of cultural competency within disaster preparedness:[11]

1. **Awareness and acceptance of difference.** Responders and survivors may be very different in their racial or ethnic identities or even speak different languages. Responders must work to become aware of any biases or stereotypes they may harbor before they can provide culturally competent care. For example, not all cultures react to stressful, emotionally trying situations in the same way.[12] Cultural competence entails becoming aware

of various culture-specific manifestations of stress to help spot people at risk of developing post-traumatic stress disorder (PTSD).

2. **Awareness of one's own cultural values.** All public health professionals, including those in communications roles, must assess their own prejudices to become aware of areas in which they may hold cultural or ethic biases. The Valuing Diversity and Self-Assessment questionnaire can be used to help identify strengths and weaknesses when working with populations of different backgrounds.[13]

3. **Understanding and managing the "dynamics of difference."** Different cultures express and interpret information in different ways. Public health professionals should be trained to gather cultural information when taking medical histories so they can provide better services. The RESPOND tool provides a way to take medical histories in diverse populations:[14]

   R – Build **rapport**
   E – **Explain** your purpose
   S – Identify **services** and elaborate
   P – Encourage individuals to be **proactive**
   O – **Offer** assistance for individuals to identify their needs
   N – **Negotiate** what is normal to help identify needs
   D – **Determine** next steps

4. **Development of cultural knowledge.** Public health professionals should become aware of the various cultural and ethnic groups in their communities and work to familiarize themselves with customs and basic language so they are better equipped to communicate during an emergency.

5. **Ability to adapt activities to fit different cultural contexts.** Public health professionals must develop the ability to adapt to the cultures they are serving. That may include modifying services as needed, such as arranging for interpreters to help in information gathering and, in the case of public health communications, information dissemination.[15]

Developing Cultural Humility

Cultural humility is defined as understanding and developing a process-oriented approach to cultural competency. The following are three factors that can guide an individual toward cultural competence and humility:

1. **A lifelong commitment to self-evaluation and self-critique.** Is a person able and willing to admit what he or she does not know? Does the person desire to learn more? There must be acceptance of the fact that one will never finish learning and must always strive for greater understanding of others.

2. **A desire to fix power imbalances where none should exist.** While public health professionals have tremendous knowledge that members of the general public do not, they must also appreciate that individuals have important information about their own backgrounds and experiences—information that must be shared in order to get to the best outcome.

3. **A desire to develop partnerships with people and groups who advocate for others.** Communities and groups can be far more effective than individuals in the push to fix power imbalances. To create positive change, there must be a collective, systemic approach to cultural humility.[16]

▶ Conclusion

The purpose of risk communication is to provide information to allow an individual, stakeholder, or whole community to make the best possible decisions about their health and well-being in the midst of a disaster. Effective public information strategies help to advance the goals of crisis and emergency risk communication. The outward flow of timely, accurate, and consistent information helps keep the public informed during an emergency event and helps engender trust of decision makers by the general public.

The responsibility for developing and disseminating coordinated and consistent messages lies with the PIO. The PIO supports the incident command structure by advising on all public information matters relating to the management of the incident. The PIO is also responsible for ensuring that messages are coordinated and integrated across jurisdictions, agencies, all levels of governments, NGOs, and the private sector. Applying the principles of crisis and emergency risk communication will ensure that all communications are distributed effectively, in a manner that is understandable by the public.

Discussion Questions

1. What is emergency public information and warning?
2. Name the responsibilities of the PIO within the ICS.
3. What is the difference between a JIS and JIC?
4. How is social media impacting communication during emergency response?

References

1. U.S. Centers for Disease Control and Prevention. Public health preparedness capabilities: national standards for state and local planning. Available at https://www.cdc.gov/phpr /readiness/00_docs/capability4.pdf. Accessed August 29, 2017.
2. Federal Emergency Management Agency. Emergency Management Institute. IS-702a. NIMS public information. Available at https://emilms.fema.gov/IS702A/. Accessed August 3, 2017.
3. U.S. Centers for Disease Control and Prevention. Crisis and emergency risk communication. Available at https://emergency.cdc.gov/cerc/resources/index.asp. Accessed August 3, 2017.
4. U.S. Centers for Disease Control and Prevention. Zika action plan summit-crisis and emergency risk communication. Available at https://www.cdc.gov/zap/pdfs/crisis-and-emergency-risk -communication.pdf. Accessed August 3, 2017.
5. Federal Communications Commission. Emergency alert system. Available at https://www .fcc.gov/general/emergency-alert-system-eas. Accessed August 15, 2017.
6. Federal Emergency Management Agency. Alerting authorities. Available at https://www .fema.gov/alerting-authorities. Accessed August 15, 2017.
7. Hughes AL, Palen L. The evolving role of the public information officer: An examination of social media in emergency management. *J Homeland Secur Emerg Manage.* 2012;9(1). doi:10.1515/1547-7355.1976. Accessed 3 September, 2017.

8. Merchant RM, Elmer S, Lurie N. Integrating social media into emergency-preparedness efforts. *New Engl J Med.* 2011;365(4):289–291.

9. U.S. Department of Homeland Security. National emergency communications plan. Available at https://www.dhs.gov/national-emergency-communications-plan. Accessed August 15, 2017.

10. Davidson TM, Price M, McCauley JL, Ruggiero KJ. Disaster impact across cultural groups: comparison of Whites, African Americans, and Latinos. *Am J Commun Psychol.* 2013;52(0): 97–105. doi:10.1007/s10464-013-9579-1.

11. U.S. Department of Health and Human Services. Cultural and linguistic competency in disaster preparedness and response fact sheet. Available at https://www.phe.gov/Preparedness /planning/abc/Pages/linguistic-facts.aspx. Accessed August 20, 2017.

12. Eisenbruch M. From post-traumatic stress disorder to cultural bereavement: diagnosis of Southeast Asian refugees. *Soc Sci Med.* 1991;33(6):673–680.

13. Rasmussen T. *The American Society for Training and Development (ASTD) Trainer's Sourcebook on Diversity.* New York, NY: McGraw-Hill; 1995.

14. U.S. Department of Health and Human Services. Think cultural health. Available at https:// cccdpcr.thinkculturalhealth.hhs.gov/PDFs/RespondHandout.pdf. Accessed August 20, 2017.

15. Tervalon M, Murray-Garcia J. Cultural humility versus cultural competence: a critical distinction in defining physician training outcomes in multicultural education. *J Health Care Poor Undeserved.* 1998;9:117–125.

16. American Psychological Association. Reflections on cultural humility. Available at http://www .apa.org/pi/families/resources/newsletter/2013/08/cultural-humility.aspx. Accessed August 20, 2017.

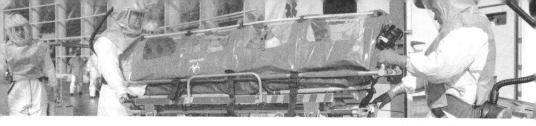

CHAPTER 12
Medical Countermeasures

LEARNING OBJECTIVES

In many large-scale public health emergencies, some type of medical countermeasure (MCM) will be needed to minimize morbidity and mortality. MCMs can include a variety of prophylactic treatments, such as vaccines, antiviral drugs, antibiotics, and antitoxins. MCM missions can be massive-scale operations that involve a complex planning and logistics process before patients can be treated, depending on the scale of the disaster in question. MCM missions can also be smaller-scale events where prophylaxis is targeted to a small, well-defined group of persons. For example, in the event of exposure to a certain infectious disease, it may be necessary to provide, over the course of several days, antivirals to a large but narrowly defined number of people who have possibly been exposed. But in the case of certain chemical attacks, it may be necessary to provide MCMs to millions of people in a matter of hours.

Public health professionals must understand the distribution chain that delivers MCMs to their door and then be able to activate plans around establishing receiving, staging, and storage (RSS) sites and points of dispensing (PODs) to provide MCMs to the public. This chapter discusses various MCMs, the methods by which they are received and dispensed during a public health incident, and the responsibilities of public health officials to:

- Identify and initiate medical countermeasure dispensing strategies
- Receive medical countermeasures
- Activate dispensing modalities
- Dispense medical countermeasures to identified population
- Report adverse events[1]

By the end of this chapter, readers should be able to:

- Understand the goals of the Strategic National Stockpile
- Describe the difference between the components of the Strategic National Stockpile
- Articulate the purpose of the establishment of POD sites
- Understand the types of MCMs that are used for various types of emergencies
- Describe several types of nonpharmaceutical interventions, and discuss why these strategies are so effective at minimizing the spread of disease

▶ Strategic National Stockpile

In 1999, the Centers for Disease Control and Prevention (CDC) created the National Pharmaceutical Stockpile to bolster readiness against potential bioterrorism threats such as anthrax, smallpox, plague, viral hemorrhagic fevers, and botulism. The purpose of the stockpile was to amass large stores of medications, including medical supplies, and place them in undisclosed, strategic locations across the country. The goal of this strategic placement was to ensure the MCMs could be delivered anywhere within the United States in less than 12 hours. In 2003, the National Pharmaceutical Stockpile was renamed the Strategic National Stockpile (SNS), and the Project BioShield Act of 2004 authorized increased spending on the SNS and placed it under the oversight of the U.S. Department of Health and Human Services. Today, the SNS contains more than $7 billion worth of medicines and medical supplies, including medications, personal protective equipment (PPE), ventilators, IV supplies, airway management supplies, and pill counting devices, among other assets.[2] It stockpiles materiel that may not be available to the general public, may not be available in the time frame in which it is needed, or may not be available in sufficient quantities to respond to a large-scale emergency.

Stockpiled Assets

The SNS includes many treatments for various illnesses and attacks. These include bacterial and viral diseases, pandemic influenza, radiation/nuclear emergencies, chemical attacks, and natural disasters.[2] The SNS components consist of materiel packaged and sustained as a two-tiered response posture. The primary component is the 12-hour push package. It serves as the first line of support to jurisdictions experiencing a large-scale public health emergency for which MCMs and medical supplies are needed for mitigation.[2] The contents of the 12-hour push package are preconfigured for rapid identification and ease of distribution. Stored in environmentally controlled and secured facilities across the country, they remain ready for deployment to reach the designated area within 12 hours of federal activation of the assets.

The second tier, more long-term component of the SNS is the vendor-managed inventory (VMI). VMI is composed of supplies and pharmaceuticals that are delivered from one or more sources, generally medical or pharmaceutical manufacturers. Because VMI are maintained by the manufacturers, they can be tailored to provide specific materiel, depending on the identified disease or cause. VMI can also be deployed as a supplement to a previously deployed 12-hour push package.[2] Maintenance of this two-tiered response capability enables the CDC to maintain a flexible and responsive posture in the supply of medical materiel following all-hazards emergencies and disasters.

Other SNS assets include CHEMPACKs and Federal Medical Stations (FMSs). CHEMPACKs are containers of nerve agent antidotes that are placed at more than 1300 strategic locations around the country. This large network of chemical countermeasures puts more than 90% of the U.S. population within 1 hour of a CHEMPACK location.[3] This high level of availability is critically important because the window of treatment for a chemical attack is narrow, generally only a few short hours. CHEMPACK locations ensure that much of the population can potentially receive treatment within a short time frame of exposure to a chemical agent.[3]

The final asset contained in the SNS is the FMS. An FMS is a non-emergency medical center that can be set up during a disaster to care for displaced persons with special health needs, whether chronic health conditions, limited mobility, or mental health issues, that cannot be addressed in a traditional shelter.[2] The healthcare capability that federal medical stations can provide is the distinguishing characteristic between an FMS and a temporary shelter. While the SNS provides these rapidly deployable, modular caches of beds, supplies, and medications, local and state officials must plan and coordinate closely with federal officials prior to the event to determine the location for setup of the stations, as well as the staffing for these assets. A team of technical specialists deploys with the FMS; however, the members of the team do not provide medical care once the stations have been activated. They provide technical assistance, training, and resource requests to ensure proper functioning and operation of the FMS. An FMS provides an additional asset that can be used when a physical location for medical surge capability is needed, or when an alternative treatment facility may be needed, separate from a hospital or other free-standing healthcare facility.

The SNS program maintains a large network of public and private partners, to ensure the public health community is prepared to develop, distribute, and dispense medical countermeasures (MCMs) following a large-scale public health emergency. As with many aspects of emergency preparedness planning, the relationships and partnerships that are developed pre-incident are the ones that are most likely to be needed when a disaster occurs. The following are examples of some of the many partners that play a critical role in the success of the SNS program:

- Federal
  - Department of Veterans' Affairs
  - Department of Defense (DOD)
  - Office of Emergency Preparedness (HHS)
  - Food and Drug Administration (HHS)
- State/local
  - Departments of Health
  - Emergency Management Agencies (EMAs)
- Private sector
  - Pharmaceutical manufacturers/vendors
  - Transportation companies

▶ Distribution Logistics: Receiving, Staging, and Storage

The SNS provides a net of protection that is nearly invisible to the general public, but the magnitude of SNS operations and the benefit to the general public are immense. When the decision is made to deploy the SNS for a large-scale incident in which the disease or agent is initially unknown, the SNS 12-hour push package is dispatched. The 12-hour push package consists of over one hundred cargo shipping containers, packed according to their contents and whether those contents are pharmaceuticals, intravenous supplies, airway management supplies, bandages, or repackaging devices. Each 12-hour push package weighs over 50 tons and can fill a wide-body aircraft.[2] **FIGURE 12-1** illustrates the size of a 12-hour push package, as

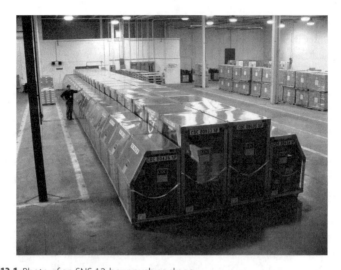

FIGURE 12-1 Photo of an SNS 12-hour push package

Reproduced from U.S. Centers for Disease Control and Prevention. Strategic National Stockpile. 12-hour Push Package. Available at: www.cdc.gov/phpr/stockpile/pushpackage.htm. Accessed: August 25, 2017.

compared to a person standing 6ft tall. Every state or receiving jurisdiction must have plans in place and the capability to receive the push package, break it down, repackage its contents, and disseminate those contents to local dispensing sites or healthcare facilities where the medications will be provided to members of the general public.

For public health, the ability to receive, stage, store, and manage SNS assets is a daunting balance of logistical elements that is outside the traditional scope of expertise for public health. Each 12-hour push package requires at least 5000 square feet of ground or floor space for proper staging. Public health planners need to locate a warehousing facility or other space with a large enough footprint to manage the assets upon their arrival. Also, logistical details must be carefully planned to determine processes for breaking down SNS assets from the bulk packaging in which the assets come, into smaller quantities that are suitable for distribution to hospitals, health clinics, or public dispensing sites. Some of the logistical details include ensuring the warehouse has the proper space, staffing, and equipment for the safe and timely breakdown of the assets, and planning truck routes for the assets to be transported from the warehousing location to the end point is key. Ensuring the availability of the proper type and size of truck and access to the routes that contain fuel stations along the way are additional details for the transportation of the assets. For any countermeasures that may have temperature sensitivities, accommodations to ensure temperature integrity can be maintained throughout the full logistics process are another important logistical consideration. Planners also need to consider the waste disposal needs of the public dispensing centers, as the assets are dispensed to the public. Improper waste disposal could lead to other public health problems, confounding the response operation. Thus, these considerations should be made within the context of the warehousing operation. Finally, during the receipt, staging, and distribution phases, public health also has to ensure tight control and security of the assets. Public health departments typically do not maintain warehousing, transportation, and security workforces. Therefore, close planning and coordination with jurisdictional and private-sector partners must be conducted to ensure capability levels for MCM management are developed.

Dispensing Operations: Points of Dispensing (PODs)

Points of dispensing (PODs) are the locations at which jurisdictions will provide MCMs to members of the public. They must be set up in locations that are easily accessible, such as near public transportation, and must be large enough to accommodate the anticipated number of patients who may visit them. Plans must consider the optimal setup of PODs to maximize efficiency and ensure that as many patients as possible can be processed through the site to receive needed treatment.

Some ways to ensure the efficiency of dispensing centers include the following:

- Setting up multiple stations to increase productivity
- Utilizing clinical staff in clinical roles and non-clinical staff in other roles
- Educating the public in groups versus one-on-one
- Eliminating repetition
- Adjusting standards of care to meet the ideal timelines within which a specific countermeasure must be taken (this can be a challenge for some clinicians)

The end goal within a POD is to "get pills into people". Therefore, critical components of the dispensing process also include proper education of the public to inform people about the need for countermeasures; collection of medical/health data to ensure proper medical screening and minimize the improper provision of any MCMs that are contraindicated for some individuals; and a plan for the management of adverse events. *Receiving, Distributing, and Dispensing Strategic National Stockpile Assets: A Guide for Preparedness* is an invaluable tool in understanding each part of the process related to receiving and dispensing MCMs from the SNS.[4]

Emergency Use Authorizations

Many of the medications available through the SNS are not generally available to the public or may not be approved by the U.S. Food and Drug Administration (FDA) for emergency use. In this situation, the Secretary of Health and Human Services is responsible for determining that such authorization is necessary in order to address the public health emergency. The Secretary can then request that the FDA Commissioner issue an Emergency Use Authorization (EUA) for the medication's use during the emergency. Only the FDA Commissioner has the authority to issue an EUA,[5] which allows jurisdictions to use specific drugs, biologics, and medical devices and to provide medications to those who need them most within the context of the public health emergency. The FDA makes this exception when such materials are necessary to diagnose, treat, or prevent a serious or life-threatening disease or condition and there are no adequate, approved, or available alternatives during an emergency. An EUA can add a layer of complexity to an MCM response, because it may contain specific circumstances under which the drug can be administered and requirements around supplemental information that must be provided to patients who receive the MCM. Jurisdictions may need to spend precious time being sure they understand all elements of an EUA, and confirm that health centers and other dispensing entities also do the same.

Pre-event Requests

While many requests for 12-hour push packs come in the wake of an unanticipated incident, it is possible for jurisdictions to request receipt of a shipment in anticipation of an event. Examples of those cases include the following:

- When there is actionable intelligence indicating an impending chemical, biological, radiological/nuclear, or large explosive attack or overwhelming public health disaster
- When an analysis of data derived from syndromic or epidemiologic surveillance indicates a coming event
- When there is a sentinel event, such as a single case of smallpox

▶ Federal Development Efforts

The threat of terrorism from chemical, biological, radiological, and nuclear (CBRN) agents remains high. However, many of the MCMs necessary to treat communities in the wake of a CBRN attack are drugs and supplies that would normally not be available in large enough quantities to address a large-scale attack, or the needed countermeasure has not yet been developed. For that reason, the federal government has passed multiple pieces of legislation to encourage the private sector to continue developing and producing life-saving medications intended to counter a CBRN attack.

Project BioShield

In 2004, Congress passed the Project Bioshield Act to establish a market to provide the federal government with new authorities related to the development, procurement, and use of MCMs against CBRN terrorism agents. The Act allocated funds to pharmaceutical companies to develop new protective drugs, as well as funds for the purchase of such drugs. It also grants the National Institutes of Health/National Institute of Allergy and Infectious Diseases the authority to expedite and simplify the solicitation, review, and award of grants and contracts for drug development.

Pandemic and All-Hazards Preparedness Act

In 2006, Congress passed the Pandemic and All-Hazards Preparedness Act (PAHPA), which established a new Assistant Secretary for Preparedness and Response (ASPR) in the Department of Health and Human Services (HHS). It also established the Biomedical Advanced Research and Development Authority (BARDA) within HHS and ASPR. BARDA is responsible for managing the development of new MCMs against CBRN threats. The BARDA Strategic Plan sets forth five overarching goals:

- **Goal 1:** An advanced development pipeline replete with medical countermeasures and platforms to address unmet public health needs, emphasizing innovation, flexibility, multi-purpose and broad spectrum application, and long-term sustainability.

- **Goal 2:** A capability base to provide enabling core services to medical countermeasure innovators.
- **Goal 3:** Agile, robust and sustainable U.S. manufacturing infrastructure capable of rapidly producing vaccines and other biologics against pandemic influenza and other emerging threats
- **Goal 4:** Responsive and nimble programs and capabilities to address novel and emerging threats
- **Goal 5:** A ready capability to develop, manufacture and facilitate distribution of medical countermeasures during public health emergencies[6]

Public Health Emergency Medical Countermeasures Enterprise

The Public Health Emergency Medical Countermeasures Enterprise (PHEMCE) was established to coordinate MCM planning and execution across federal organizations in charge of protecting the civilian population from potential adverse health impacts. The PHEMCE is led by ASPR and includes three primary HHS internal agency partners: the CDC, the FDA, and the National Institutes of Health (NIH). In addition, there are several interagency partners: the Department of Defense (DoD), the U.S. Department of Veterans Affairs (VA), the Department of Homeland Security (DHS), and the U.S. Department of Agriculture (USDA).

The PHEMCE mission includes the following:

- **Requirements setting.** PHEMCE must establish requirements for civilian medical countermeasures based on many factors, including threat and risk assessments.
- **Early-stage research.** NIH, [DoD and USDA] conduct and support basic research to better understand threats of civilian public health concern.
- **Advanced development/manufacturing.** ASPR/BARDA is the lead PHEMCE partner supporting advanced development and scale-up of manufacturing capacity for medical countermeasures.
- **Regulatory science management.** PHEMCE conducts regulatory science to facilitate MCM development, regulatory assessment, and use.
- **Procurement/inventory management/stockpiling.** PHEMCE oversees the procurement of MCMs and their associated inventory management, including stockpiling.
- **Response planning, policy, guidance and communication.** The CDC and ASPR coordinate the development of federal response plans, policy, guidance and communication, and develop clinical utilization and allocation strategies.
- **Deployment/distribution/dispensing/administration.** The CDC and ASPR coordinate interactions with state, local, tribal, territorial (SLTT), and private entities to provide timely and effective deployment, distribution, dispensing, and administration.
- **Monitoring/evaluation/assessment.** The CDC and FDA monitor safety and performance of deployed MCMs during and after an emergency response.[7]

PHEMCE represents a multiagency, multidisciplinary policy and implementation process. The level of leadership represented within the enterprise is indicative of the importance of ensuring the availability of appropriate MCMs to protect the citizens of the United States from all hazards emergencies and disasters. PHEMCE requirements are set such that development and acquisition of countermeasures meet specific preparedness goals, as set forth by BARDA, within the U.S. Department of Health and Human Services.[8]

▶ Alternate MCM Delivery Methods

In 2009, President Barack Obama signed Presidential Executive Order 13527. This executive order put forth a policy requirement for the U.S. government "to plan and prepare for the timely provision of medical countermeasures to the American people in the event of a biological attack in the United States through a rapid Federal response in coordination with State, local, territorial, and tribal governments."[9] This policy sought to "mitigate illness and prevent death; sustain critical infrastructure; and to complement and supplement State, local, territorial, and tribal government medical countermeasure distribution capacity."[9] The primary impetus behind the order was to ensure an appropriate federal-level response to a biological attack.

However, another component of the order recognized the important role that state and local jurisdictions would play in a biological attack, and thus called upon state and local jurisdictions to develop alternate distribution methods that could offer faster, less restrictive delivery of MCMs to the public. Some examples of alternate dispensing methods include the following:

- Delivery via U.S. Postal Service
- Home MedKits
- "Closed" PODs (e.g., for large employers with medical infrastructure that can support at-work distribution to employees)

Jurisdictions had autonomy to determine whether or not any of these alternative methods for MCM countermeasure dispensing would be acceptable within their jurisdictions or if they would further complicate any local or state MCM distribution and dispensing efforts. The postal model concept entailed the delivery of antibiotic medications through the postal service, with delivery being made by a postal worker in the same manner traditional mail is delivered. This model was found to be a viable option in many jurisdictions, but certainly not all. Some large cities were unable to implement the postal model because postal workers demanded 1:1 police escorts. With less police officers than postal workers, this approach never took off in these jurisdictions.

The Home MedKits option was another alternative strategy that was also short-lived. This strategy entailed prepositioning antibiotic medications and PPE in the homes of first responders for use by themselves and their family members, in the event of a biological release. The problem with Home MedKits came with uncertainty as to whether households could properly store medications and supplies to ensure their integrity, as well as the realization that once the medications contained within the kits expired, they would be expensive to replace.[10]

The concept of closed PODs was the more successful of the alternative method models. Partnerships with private-sector businesses have enabled health officials to plan for the implementation of closed PODs, PODs that are only open to employees and family members for the companies holding the closed PODs. These facilities operate in the same manner a traditional, open, public POD would, with the exception of being limited to specific employees. Closed PODs provide an opportunity for large segments of the population to receive their medications, outside of the general public being cared for by local officials, thus minimizing the crowding and logistical burden in the open PODs.

▶ Community Mitigation

In some public health crises—particularly in the case of an emerging infectious disease—the best MCM to treat a population may not be immediately available for weeks or months. For example, a new strain of pandemic flu could spread unchecked until a viable vaccine is developed, distributed, and dispensed. In these cases, it will be necessary to implement nonpharmaceutical interventions (NPIs). At the individual level, those NPIs can be as simple as frequently washing hands, covering coughs and sneezes, staying home when sick, and routinely disinfecting surfaces. At the community level, we refer to community mitigation as the actions that communities may take to decrease or prevent their exposure to disease. As a first line of defense against certain infectious diseases, community mitigation tactics can decrease transmission substantially.

Community mitigation may include any or all of the following interventions:

- **Isolation and treatment** (as appropriate) with influenza antiviral medications of all persons with confirmed or probable pandemic influenza. Isolation may occur in the home or healthcare setting, depending on the severity of an individual's illness and the current capacity of the healthcare infrastructure.
- **Voluntary home quarantine** of members of households with confirmed or probable influenza cases and consideration of combining this intervention with the prophylactic use of antiviral medications, providing that sufficient quantities of effective medications exist and that a feasible means of distributing them is in place.
- **Dismissal of students** from school (including public and private schools as well as colleges and universities) and school-based activities and closure of childcare programs, coupled with protecting children and teenagers through social distancing in the community to achieve reductions of out-of-school social contacts and community mixing.
- Use of **social distancing measures** to reduce contact between adults in the community and workplace, including cancellation of large public gatherings and alteration of workplace environments and schedules to decrease social density and preserve a healthy workplace to the greatest extent possible without disrupting essential services.[11]

These interventions can be quite large in scope, and implementing them in a timely and organized manner requires public health professionals to plan for them carefully. Plans should include the conditions under which each of these measures becomes necessary and how these measures will be communicated to the affected populations and agencies who will enforce them. Agencies, communities, schools, and workplaces must also prepare for the consequences of these interventions, such as childcare accommodations for working parents when school closure has been implemented as an NPI. While difficult to plan for, NPIs are effective measures for minimizing the spread of disease.

▶ Conclusion

MCMs provide life-saving medical interventions following an event of public health significance. Whether the required intervention is an oral medication, a vaccine, the proper equipment required to administer such medications, or a location to provide for the medical/mental/behavioral health of victims, the federal government's capacity for provision of these interventions via the SNS is relatively unknown to the general public but highly beneficial to the protection of the public. The management of the assets contained within the SNS requires significant planning and coordination by public health officials. The high degree of logistical considerations related to the management of the assets through both the distribution and dispensing processes necessitates inclusion of multiple emergency management partners throughout the planning and response. It is imperative that public health officials work carefully with their partners, including the private sector, to ensure all logistical elements are included in the plan and tested through drills and exercises to ensure the MCM mission can be met when necessary.

Discussion Questions

1. What is the purpose of the SNS?
2. Does the SNS contain materials for only certain types of emergencies, or all-hazards emergencies?
3. What is the amount of floor space needed for proper receipt and staging of the SNS? Why is such a large amount of space needed for this function?
4. Name three alternative dispensing methods for MCMs. Are any of these methods currently viable for implementation? Why or why not?
5. Name four NPIs that can be effective in minimizing the spread of disease. In your opinion, why are these measures so successful?

References

1. Centers for Disease Control and Prevention. Public health preparedness capabilities: national standards for state and local planning. 2011;71. https://www.cdc.gov/phpr/readiness/00_docs/DSLR_capabilities_July.pdf.
2. Centers for Disease Control and Prevention. Stockpile products. Available at https://www.cdc.gov/phpr/stockpile/products.htm. Accessed August 25, 2017.
3. Centers for Disease Control and Prevention. CDC's CHEMPACK Program—The Stockpile that may protect you from a chemical attack. *Public Health Matters Blog.* Available at https://blogs.cdc.gov/publichealthmatters/2015/02/cdcs-chempack-program-the-stockpile-that-may-protect-you-from-a-chemical-attack/. Accessed August 26, 2017.
4. Centers for Disease Control and Prevention. Receiving, distributing, and dispensing strategic national stockpile assets: a guide for preparedness. Available at http://www.ema.ohio.gov/Documents/Plans/ReceivingDistributingandDispensingStrategicNationalStockpileAssets_%20AGuidetoPreparedness_Version11.pdf. Accessed August 26, 2017.
5. Nightingale SL, Prasher JM, Simonson S. Emergency Use Authorization (EUA) to enable use of needed products in civilian and military emergencies, United States. *Emerging Infect Dis.* 2007;13(7):1046. doi:10.3201/eid1307.061188.
6. U.S. Department of Health and Human Services. Barda unveils path forward in the BARDA strategic plans. Available at https://www.phe.gov/about/barda/Pages/2011barda-stratplan.aspx. Last Reviewed April 27, 2015. Accessed September 1, 2017.

7. U.S. Department of Health and Human Services. PHEMCE mission components. Available at https://www.phe.gov/Preparedness/mcm/phemce/Pages/mission.aspx. Last Reviewed February 27, 2015. Accessed September 1, 2017.

8. U.S. Department of Health and Human Services. About the PHEMCE. Available at https://www.medicalcountermeasures.gov/phemce.aspx. Accessed August 29, 2017.

9. Executive Order 13527. Establishing federal capability for the timely provision of medical countermeasures following a biological attack. Homeland Security Digital Library. Available at https://www.hsdl.org/?abstract&did=30694. Accessed September 1, 2017.

10. Institute of Medicine Forum on Medical and Public Health Preparedness for Catastrophic Events. Medical Countermeasures Dispensing: Emergency Use Authorization and the Postal Model, Workshop Summary. Washington, DC: National Academies Press (US); 2010. *The Postal Model*. Available at https://www.ncbi.nlm.nih.gov/books/NBK53124/.

11. Centers for Disease Control and Prevention. Interim pre-pandemic planning guidance: community strategy for pandemic influenza mitigation in the United States—early, targeted, layered use of nonpharmaceutical interventions. Available at https://www.cdc.gov/flu/pandemic-resources/pdf/community_mitigation-sm.pdf. Accessed August 30, 2017.

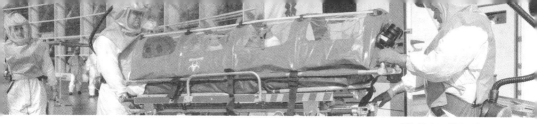

CHAPTER 13

Medical Surge

LEARNING OBJECTIVES

Large-scale disasters and emergencies, such as mass-casualty events, infectious disease outbreaks, and bioterrorism attacks, will likely place significant demands on hospitals and healthcare systems. Depending on the size, scale, and scope of the specific emergency and the capabilities of individual facilities, hospitals may be faced with the need to care for a greater number of patients than is typical from their daily census. Medical surge refers to "the ability to provide adequate medical evaluation and care during events that exceed the limits of the normal medical infrastructure of an affected community".[1] It also includes the ability of the hospital or healthcare system to survive the impact of the hazard and maintain or rapidly recover operations that were compromised. There are two unique considerations that make up medical surge: surge capacity and surge capability. Surge capacity is "the ability to manage the sudden influx of patients, beyond normal capacity, and having the space, staff, and other resources to effectively provide care. Surge capability refers to the ability to care for patients who have specialized medical care needs. These specialized needs will likely be related to the disaster itself, but could also be the result of an already known medical condition that is exacerbated by the disaster".[2]

Recent natural disasters have tested the medical surge capability of several hospitals and healthcare systems across the United States. Disasters such as the Joplin, Missouri, tornado of 2011 in which 158 people were killed and 1150 were injured; and Hurricane Katrina in 2005 in which 1245 were killed and thousands had to be rescued are two examples. The 2009–2010 H1N1 outbreak, the Ebola response of 2014–2015, and the subsequent Zika response in 2015, were infectious disease emergencies that also tested the medical surge abilities of hospitals and healthcare systems across the United States. As this book was being prepared for publication, Hurricane Harvey was ravaging Houston, Texas, and the Gulf Coast. The full degree of damage and destruction following Hurricane Harvey will not be known for some time, but the images of medically fragile infants being evacuated from Houston-area hospitals and elderly residents sitting waist high in flooded nursing homes give us an indication that the medical surge needs and overall response needs are significant, likely beyond what was experienced during Hurricane Katrina, which struck the same region some 20 years ago. This chapter explores the challenges faced by public health and the healthcare system to develop and maintain the capability to provide medical care during and after emergencies and disasters. By the end of this chapter, readers should be able to:

- Define medical surge and articulate the importance of developing medical surge capability
- Understand the role of healthcare coalitions (HCCs) in developing healthcare preparedness and response capability
- Articulate the importance of ensuring ethical standards are employed in preparedness planning
- Understand the concept of mutual aid and how assistance can be critical in ensuring medical surge
- Identify federal resources that are available for aid in mass emergency situations

▶ Medical Surge Management

Because medical surge entails, by definition, circumstances that are highly unusual, planning for and managing these events require special capabilities that cannot be met by a single entity. Multiple entities must work together to build a single, unified response plan and be prepared to carry it out cooperatively during a surge. In recent years, healthcare coalitions (HCCs) have become an important mechanism for the coordinated planning that is required to ensure the medical needs of disaster victims and the surge needs of healthcare systems can be met in the midst of crises situations. The call for the establishment of health care coalitions represents an evolution from a focus on individual facility preparedness to a focus on preparedness of the full healthcare system, including public health and emergency management, to respond to disasters and emergencies.

▶ Healthcare System Preparedness

Healthcare system preparedness is a core capability that must be developed in jurisdictions across the country to ensure appropriate levels of medical surge management in response to large-scale emergencies and disasters. Healthcare system preparedness efforts are funded by the U.S. Department of Health and Human Services, Office of the Assistant Secretary for Preparedness and Response (ASPR). Allocating funding to 62 awardees across the United States, ASPR "leads the country in preparing for, responding to, and recovering from the adverse health effects of emergencies and disasters."[2(pg.5)] ASPR's "Hospital Preparedness Program (HPP) is the only source of federal funding for health care delivery system readiness, intended to improve patient outcomes, minimize the need for federal and supplemental state resources during emergencies, and enable rapid recovery. HPP prepares the health care delivery system to save lives through the development of health care coalitions (HCCs) that incentivize diverse and often competitive health care organizations with differing priorities and objectives to work together."[2(pg.5)]

FIGURE 13-1 displays the funding ASPR has awarded for HPP awardees since the inception of the cooperative agreement grant program in 2002.

Hospital Preparedness Program (HPP)
cooperative agreement funding allocations

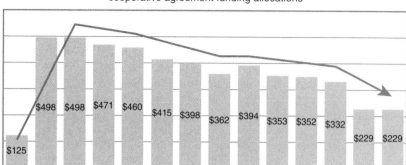

FIGURE 13-1 HPP cooperative agreement funding allocations

Data from U.S. Department of Health and Human Services. Office of the Assistant Secretary for Preparedness and Response.

▶ Healthcare Coalitions

Complicating a medical surge scenario is the fact that many patients, depending on the nature of the disaster, may have unusual or highly specialized needs. To handle an influx of these patients in a large-scale disaster, medical and public health officials will need to work in close collaboration and create coalitions. HCCs are a critical component of medical surge management both during the planning stage and in the midst of an emergency. An HCC is a collaborative network of individual healthcare and response organizations (e.g., hospitals, emergency medical services [EMS], emergency management organizations, public health agencies, etc.) in a defined geographic location, that work collaboratively to develop healthcare delivery system preparedness and response capabilities. HCCs serve as multiagency coordinating groups that support and integrate with Emergency Support Function 8 (ESF-8) activities in the context of Incident Command System (ICS) responsibilities.[2] Public health planners have the responsibility of forming HCCs with participation from a variety of public- and private-sector partners, including the following:

- Hospitals and healthcare providers
- Public health
- Emergency management
- Emergency medical services
- Public safety
- Long-term care providers
- Mental/behavioral health providers
- Private entities associated with health care (hospital associations)
- Public/private labs
- Specialty providers (dialysis, pediatrics, women's health, stand-alone surgery, urgent care)
- Support service providers (blood banks, pharmacies, poison control)
- Community health centers
- Primary care providers

- Tribal health care
- Federal entities (VA hospitals, Indian Health Service (IHS) facilities, DOD facilities)

HCC members will work together to coordinate preparedness efforts that involve member organizations and assist in the development of local and state emergency operations plans that address the medical surge needs of the jurisdiction. This planning closely resembles the planning process traditionally undertaken by public health emergency planners, utilizing the Preparedness Cycle, and entails identifying healthcare system risks and vulnerabilities, prioritizing healthcare assets and essential services within a healthcare delivery area or region, assessing available resources, coordinating training and exercise activities to test plans, ensuring compliance with regulatory rules (i.e., accrediting requirements), and working together to develop plans that specifically address the needs of at-risk populations.

▶ Management Systems

HCCs will require systems that can effectively manage medical and health response (**FIGURE 13-2**). The Medical Surge Capacity and Capability (MSCC) Management System describes a system of interdisciplinary coordination based on the use of the ICS. It emphasizes responsibility rather than authority for assigning key response functions and advocates a management-by-objectives approach (**FIGURE 13-3**). In doing so, the MSCC Management System describes a National Incident Management System–compatible framework of coordination and integration across six tiers of response:

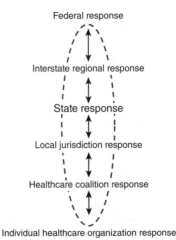

Public health and medical response
management across the intergovernmental
and public-private divides

Federal response

Interstate regional response

State response

Local jurisdiction response

Healthcare coalition response

Individual healthcare organization response

FIGURE 13-2 Public health and medical response management across the intergovernmental and public–private divides

Data from U.S. Department of Health and Human Services. Medical Surge Capacity and Capability Handbook. Available at: www.phe.gov /preparedness/planning/mscc/handbook/documents/mscc080626.pdf. Accessed: August 21, 2017.

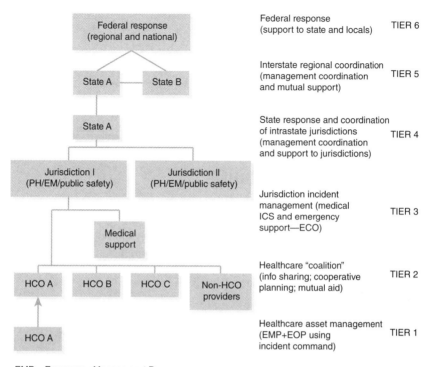

EMP = Emergency Management Program
EOP = Emergency Operations Plan
PH   = Public Health
EM   = Emergency Management
HCO = Healthcare Organization

FIGURE 13-3 MSCC Management System

Data from U.S. Department of Health and Human Services. Medical Surge Capacity and Capability Handbook. Available at: www.phe.gov
/preparedness/planning/mscc/handbook/documents/mscc080626.pdf. Accessed: August 21, 2017.

- Tier 1: Management of individual healthcare assets. A well-defined ICS to collect and process information, to develop incident plans, and to manage decisions is essential to maximize MSCC.
- Tier 2: Management of an HCC. The HCC provides a central integration mechanism for information sharing and management coordination among healthcare assets.
- Tier 3: Jurisdiction incident management. A jurisdiction's ICS integrates healthcare assets with other response disciplines to provide the structure and support needed to maximize MSCC.
- Tier 4: Management of state response. State government participates in medical incident response across a range of capacities, depending on the specific event. The state may be the lead incident command authority, it may provide support to incidents managed at the jurisdictional (Tier 3) level, or it may coordinate multijurisdictional incident response.
- Tier 5: Interstate regional management coordination. Incident management coordination between affected states ensures consistency in regional response through coordinated incident planning, enhances information exchange between interstate jurisdictions, and maximizes MSCC through interstate mutual aid and other support.

- Tier 6: Federal support to state, tribal, and jurisdiction management. Effective management processes at the state (Tier 4) and jurisdiction (Tier 3) levels facilitate the request, receipt, and integration of federal public health and medical resources to maximize MSCC.[3]

An understanding of the ICS is integral to the development of medical surge capability. For more in-depth information on ICS, see Chapter 1: What Is Public Health Preparedness? and Chapter 10: Multiagency Coordination Systems, Information Sharing, and Interoperability.

▶ Critical Responsibilities

Medical surge management begins with the collection and analysis of health data to assess and fully understand the situation. These data will be used to define the incident, identify needs, and allocate available personnel and other resources that can come from EMS, fire departments, law enforcement, public health, medical providers, and public works departments. In addition, other critical management responsibilities during a medical surge include the following:

- Ensuring adequate patient care
- Promoting medical system resiliency
- Ensuring responder safety
- Managing information management
- Coordinating diverse operating systems
- Resolving intergovernmental issues
- Supporting medical assets
- Addressing time constraints
- Incorporating medical and public health assets into public safety response[3]

▶ Crisis Standards of Care

In public health events that cause a medical surge, healthcare entities may be forced to adjust their normal standards of care in order to provide care to a large influx of patients. In a catastrophic event that causes damage to buildings and infrastructure, a healthcare facility's ability to provide the optimal level of care may be impacted by resource constraints. Each of these situations was present during Hurricane Katrina in 2005 and the 2009–2010 H1N1 outbreak. As a result of these two events, in 2009, ASPR requested the Institute of Medicine (IOM) convene a panel of experts to develop guidance for crisis standards of care (CSC) to be employed in disaster situations.[4] As seen in **FIGURE 13-4**, the framework promotes standards that are based on a foundation of ethical considerations in the context of a jurisdiction's legal authority and environment. CSC planning also requires extensive education, information sharing, and engagement of the public and healthcare provider communities. Hospitals, public health, out-of-hospital care providers, EMS, and emergency management officials must all be involved in the planning, under the authority of local, state, and federal governments. The change in care standards becomes justified when a disaster or emergency renders a healthcare system incapable of meeting normal standards. CSC is based on the concept that it

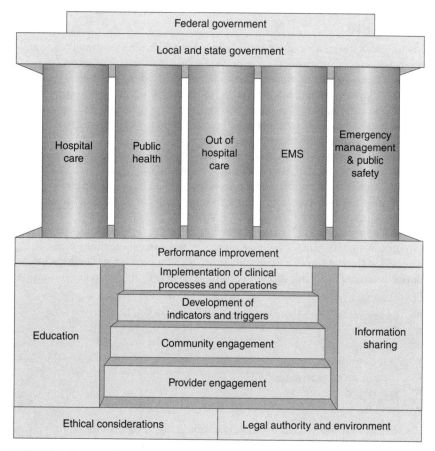

FIGURE 13-4 A systems framework for catastrophic disaster response

Reproduced from National Academies of Sciences, Engineering and Medicine. Crisis Standards of Care: A Systens Framework for Catastrophic Disaster Response. Available at: www.nationalacademies.org/hmd/Reports/2012/Crisis-Standards-of-Care-A-Systems -Framework-for-Catastrophic-Disaster-Response.aspx. Accessed: August 21, 2017.

is better to provide adequate care to all people than to provide exceptional care to some and no care to others.

▶ Mutual Aid and Federal Assistance

All incidents are local, and most incidents are managed completely at the local level, although some incidents may require state, regional, or federal assistance. Therefore, in planning for meeting the medical surge needs of the community, jurisdictions should identify and agree to the resources that may be available from neighboring communities or other levels of government during an incident. While mutual aid will be available from neighboring communities during some events, it is important for emergency planners to consider the fact that for a large-scale event that impacts multiple states, state or federal assistance may be the only option available for assistance.

Mutual Aid

Mutual aid agreements are agreements among neighboring communities, emergency responders, or jurisdictions to provide assistance to one another, when possible, during emergency responses. These agreements facilitate a jurisdiction's ability to offer supplies, equipment, personnel, information, or other resources across political boundaries during an emergency response.[5] Formal mutual aid agreements should be developed and formalized during the planning phase to ensure assistance is available during the response phase.

Once an incident does occur, immediate actions, including the execution of emergency plans and actions to support short-term recovery, must be taken to save lives, protect property and the environment, and meet basic human needs. Thus, planning for resource and supply shortages in advance can ensure that jurisdictions are able to fulfill the mission of protecting citizens.

Additionally, states play a key role in coordinating resources and capabilities throughout the state and obtaining resources and capabilities from other states. The role of the state government in response is to supplement local efforts before, during, and after incidents. A state's resources available in an emergency include the following:

- Emergency management and homeland security agencies
- State police
- Health agencies
- Transportation agencies
- Incident management teams
- Specialized teams
- National Guard

The federal government maintains a wide array of capabilities and resources that can assist state governments in responding to incidents and ensuring appropriate medical surge capability. When an incident exceeds or is anticipated to exceed state, tribal, or local resources, the federal government may provide resources and capabilities to support the state response.

National Disaster Medical System

The National Disaster Medical System (NDMS) is a collaboration between the Departments of Health and Human Services, Homeland Security, and Veterans Affairs. It provides a federal disaster response to state and local jurisdictions in the form of personnel, supplies, and equipment; helps move patients away from disaster sites and to safe, unaffected areas; and provides medical care at member hospitals. NDMS is intended for action in domestic emergencies, but partner organizations have also responded jointly to international disasters, such as the 2010 Haiti earthquake.[6]

Disaster Medical Assistance Team

A Disaster Medical Assistance Team (DMAT) is a group of professional and paraprofessional medical personnel, supported by logistical and administrative staff, that helps to provide medical care during a disaster.[7] DMATs are a federal resource that can deploy to disaster sites with sufficient supplies and equipment to sustain themselves for 72 hours while providing medical care at a fixed or temporary medical care site, such as a Federal Medical Station (refer to Chapter 12, SNS components). The goal of a DMAT is to operate at disaster sites and staging facilities until other federal resources can arrive. DMAT members are licensed and certified to perform a number of healthcare functions in a disaster situation, including but not limited to triage, preparing patients for evacuation, as well as providing medical care.

Disaster Mortuary Operational Response Team

A Disaster Mortuary Operational Response Team (DMORT) is a federal asset that deploys to a disaster area to assist with the victim identification and mortuary services aspects of a response where there are a large number of fatalities. Composed of private citizens who provide technical assistance in identifying and processing deceased victims of a disaster, team members can represent a variety of relevant fields and may be funeral directors, medical examiners, coroners, pathologists, forensic anthropologists, medical records technicians and transcribers, fingerprint specialists, forensic odontologists, dental assistants, X-ray technicians, mental health specialists, computer professionals, administrative support staff, and security and investigative personnel.[8] Similar to a DMAT, activation of a team temporarily identifies all members as intermittent federal employees, so their certifications and licenses are valid within all 50 U.S. states.

▶ Volunteer Management

During an emergency that requires a medical surge beyond the scope of a healthcare system's normal capabilities, volunteers can fill critical gaps in service delivery. "Volunteer management is the ability to coordinate the identification, recruitment, registration, credential verification, training, and engagement of those volunteers to support the jurisdictional public health agency's response to public health events."[1(pg.133)]

While many people will spontaneously volunteer out of goodwill once an emergency occurs, healthcare systems and patients would be better served by proactively identifying and registering volunteers in the planning phase. By approaching volunteer management in this manner, planners and responders will be better equipped to develop a clear picture of how many volunteer resources will be available, under what circumstances they should be mobilized, what particular skills they may be able to contribute, and any potential legal liability issues involved in utilizing volunteers. Several mechanisms already exist for identifying available volunteer resources.

Emergency System for Advance Registration of Volunteer Health Professionals

The Emergency System for Advance Registration of Volunteer Health Professionals (ESAR-VHP) is a network of state-based registries of health professionals. This network is established prior to an event so these professionals may be called on and put to work in a more efficient manner. The ESAR-VHP "verifies volunteers' identities, licenses, credentials, accreditations, and hospital privileges in advance, saving critical time in a disaster".[9]

Medical Reserve Corps

The Medical Reserve Corps (MRC) is a national network for local volunteers to register in advance of emergencies. Public health officials can use these options to recruit, identify, train, and call up volunteers.[10] MRC units are community based and function as a way to organize and utilize local volunteers who want to donate their time and expertise to prepare for and respond to emergencies and promote healthy living throughout the year. MRC volunteers can include physicians, nurses, pharmacists, dentists, veterinarians, and epidemiologists, but nonmedical community members can also fill important roles, as there is often a need for interpreters, chaplains, office workers, legal advisors, and others during a crisis.

Community Emergency Response Team

The Community Emergency Response Team (CERT) program trains volunteers in basic disaster response skills, such as fire safety, basic medical operations, light search and rescue, psychology, and team organization and disaster medical operations. A CERT is an effective way to mobilize nonmedical volunteers who can be relied upon to assist in basic operations in the event of a disaster, freeing up medical and public health professionals to focus their attention on more complex tasks. There are currently more than 2700 CERT programs in the United States, and more than 600,000 individuals have been trained as CERT volunteers since the program's inception in 1993.[11]

▶ Responder Safety and Health

Often when emergency responders arrive at the scene of a disaster, threats and dangers may be present that can affect survivors and responders alike. The disaster may be ongoing, such as in the case of a chemical spill or radiological emergency. A disaster may also create secondary conditions that pose new risks. For example, in the aftermath of September 11, responders were in danger of air pollution from particulate matter and physical injury from cleanup at the site of the collapsed Twin Towers. In both scenarios, public health planners had the responsibility to ensure, to the highest degree possible, the safety and health of those who have come to the community's aid. Specific planning must be conducted to ensure responder safety and health at all times when responding to all-hazards disasters.

Responder Safety and Health is defined as "the ability to protect public health agency staff responding to an incident and the ability to support the health and safety needs of hospital and medical facility personnel, if requested."[1(pg.127)] "This capability consists of the ability to identify responder safety and health risks, identify safety and personal protective equipment (PPE) needs, coordinate with partners to facilitate risk-specific safety and health training, and monitor responder safety and health actions".[1(pg.127)]

When creating plans, public health planners must identify all medical risks, environmental exposures, and mental/behavioral health risks that could affect fellow responders in the course of a disaster response. This process should be done in cooperation with partner agencies and should be based on a jurisdictional risk assessment. After planners have identified all of the potential threats, they should consult subject matter experts (SMEs) to create recommendations that will be incorporated into safety plans. Within the incident command structure, the designated safety officer is charged with ensuring that the safety plan is implemented during the emergency response and will advise the incident commander and operations section chief on issues related to the health and safety of responding personnel.[12]

▶ Personal Protective Equipment

The most obvious form of assuring responder health and safety is through the acquisition and maintenance of PPE for the potential hazards and threats to which responders could be exposed to during an emergency event.[13] Recommendations for responder safety and health should include any PPE responders will need or protective actions they must take to effectively fulfill their roles. There are four categories of PPE based on the level of protection each affords:

- **Level A:** Provides the greatest level of skin, respiratory, and eye protection. Can include items such as a self-contained breathing apparatus (SCBA), boots, overalls, hard hats, disposable protective suits, and gloves.
- **Level B:** Used when the highest level of respiratory protection is necessary but a lesser level of skin protection is needed.
- **Level C:** Used when concentrations and types of airborne substances are known and the criteria for using air-purifying respirators are met.
- **Level D:** Consists of a work uniform affording minimal protection to prevent nuisance contamination only.[14]

▶ Emergency Responder Health Monitoring and Surveillance

When responders are exposed to hazardous conditions during emergency situations, it is important to ensure there is a process in place to monitor the health of responders after the emergency has ended. The purpose of this ongoing monitoring is to continue to assess the health and safety of responders to identify any concerns or conditions that may arise after the disaster. The Emergency Responder Health Monitoring and Surveillance framework enables the collection of data about responder safety and health in an organized, systematic manner and can help public health professionals better plan for responder protection in future events.[15] It includes registering and credentialing, health screening predeployment, training, health monitoring during an event, and postdeployment tracking of responder health over time.

▶ Mental Health

While much of the focus during a disaster response will be on the immediate physical risks that threaten responders, it is equally important to identify the mental and behavioral health risks and to address these risks prior to, during, and after an incident. Responders may experience a broad range of mental health consequences, as a result of exposure to extraordinarily traumatizing situations.[16] The psychological effects of this exposure can take days or weeks to set in. They may cause new mental health episodes or exacerbate existing conditions. During prolonged response efforts, resources will need to be available to mitigate mental health situations that are initiated when responders are fulfilling their response roles. Psychological first aid (PFA) is a critical tool not only for patients but also for responders to protect against long-term effects due to direct exposure to traumatic events.

▶ Conclusion

Major emergencies and disasters will severely challenge the ability of healthcare systems to adequately care for large numbers of patients (surge capacity) and/or victims with unusual or highly specialized medical needs (surge capability). The goal of medical surge capability is to ensure the ability of hospitals and healthcare systems to accommodate sudden increases in patient load due to such emergencies. Close coordination among public health and medical response partners to ensure a systematic approach to the organization and coordination of response assets and resources is also critical to effective medical surge management.

A range of resources support medical surge efforts. HCCs are important networks for coordinating assets and resources in a community in advance of an emergency requiring medical surge capability. Volunteers are an integral part of the management of an emergency requiring surge medical operations. The MRC and CERT are two valuable resources for identifying volunteers to augment the health and medical response.

Discussion Questions

1. What is medical surge? Why is the development of medical surge capability so important for emergency planners?
2. What is an HCC? List the partners/disciplines that should be included in the membership of a local HCC.
3. Explain the CSC framework.
4. What are two resources local planners have for identifying volunteer responders? What is the system that might be used for the advanced registration and credentialing of healthcare volunteers?
5. What level of PPE is needed when the highest degree of respiratory protection is needed, but a lower level of skin protection can be used?
6. What is the difference between a DMAT and a DMORT team? Identify the types of situations for which each of these teams might be deployed.

References

1. Centers for Disease Control and Prevention. Public health preparedness capabilities: national standards for state and local planning. Available at https://www.cdc.gov/phpr /readiness/00_docs/DSLR_capabilities_July.pdf. Accessed August 21, 2017.
2. U.S. Department of Health and Human Services. 2017–2022 Healthcare preparedness and response capabilities. Available at https://www.phe.gov/Preparedness/planning/hpp /reports/Documents/2017-2022-healthcare-pr-capablities.pdf. Accessed August 21, 2017.

3. U.S. Department of Health and Human Services. Medical surge capacity and capability handbook: a management system for integrating medical and health resources during large-scale emergencies. Available at https://www.phe.gov/Preparedness/planning/hpp/reports/Pages/default.aspx. Accessed August 21, 2017.

4. Institute of Medicine. Guidance for establishing crisis standards of care for use in disaster situations. Report Brief. Available at http://www.nationalacademies.org/hmd/~/media/Files/Report%20Files/2009/DisasterCareStandards/Standards%20of%20Care%20report%20brief%20FINAL.pdf. Accessed August 21, 2017.

5. Stier DD, Goodman RA. Mutual aid agreements: essential legal tools for public health preparedness and response. *Am J Public Health.* 2007;97(Suppl 1):S62–S68. doi:10.2105/AJPH.2006.101626.

6. U.S. Department of Health and Human Services. National disaster medical system. Available at https://www.phe.gov/Preparedness/responders/ndms/Pages/default.aspx. Accessed August 21, 2017.

7. U.S. Department of Health and Human Services. Disaster Medical Assistance Team. Available at https://www.phe.gov/Preparedness/responders/ndms/teams/Pages/dmat.aspx. Accessed August 21, 2017.

8. U.S. Department of Health and Human Services. Disaster Mortuary Operational Response Teams. Available at https://www.phe.gov/Preparedness/responders/ndms/teams/Pages/dmort.aspx. Accessed August 21, 2017.

9. U.S. Department of Health and Human Services. The emergency system for advance registration of volunteer health professionals. Available at https://www.phe.gov/esarvhp/pages/about.aspx. Accessed August 21, 2017.

10. U. S. Department of Health and Human Services. Medical Reserve Corps. Available at https://mrc.hhs.gov/pageViewFldr/About. Accessed August 21, 2017.

11. U.S. Department of Homeland Security. Community Emergency Response Teams. Available at https://www.ready.gov/community-emergency-response-team. Accessed August 21, 2017.

12. Federal Emergency Management Agency. IS-100b. Introduction to the incident command system training course. Available at https://emilms.fema.gov/is100b/index.htm. Accessed August 21, 2017.

13. U.S. Department of Labor, Occupational Safety and Health Administration. Personal protective equipment. Available at https://www.osha.gov/Publications/osha3151.pdf. Accessed August 21, 2017.

14. U.S. Department of Labor, Occupational Safety and Health Administration. Regulations (Standards—29 CFR, Part 1910). Occupational Safety and Health Standards. Available at https://www.osha.gov/pls/oshaweb/owadisp.show_document?p_table=standards&p_id=9767. Accessed August 21, 2017.

15. U.S. Centers for Disease Control and Prevention. Emergency responder health monitoring and surveillance. Available at https://www.cdc.gov/niosh/erhms/default.html. Accessed August 21, 2017.

16. Benedek DM, Fullerton C, Ursano RJ. First responders: Mental health consequences of natural and human-made disasters for public health and public safety workers. *Annu Rev Public Health.* 2007;28:55–68.

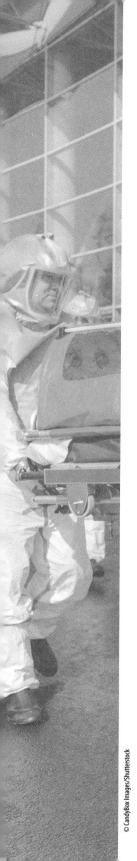

© CandyBox Images/Shutterstock

PART V

Conclusion

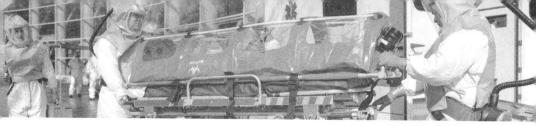

© CandyBox Images/Shutterstock

CHAPTER 14

Leadership for the Future of Public Health Preparedness

LEARNING OBJECTIVES

Emergencies and crises can unfold quickly and unpredictably, often with catastrophic results. Organizations that fail to plan will fail to uphold their mission—and it is the responsibility of the leader to ensure that does not happen. It is impossible to prepare for every event, but a prepared leader plans relentlessly, then responds with flexibility and a calm resolve, regardless of the situation.

Let's be clear: leading is very different than managing. Leaders must be visionary. That is, they must be able to develop a vision and convince others to share in that vision. This quality could not be more important than it is with leaders who are charged with leading the response to public health emergencies and disasters. Strong, effective leaders are critical to building and sustaining the public health infrastructure. By the end of this chapter, readers should be able to:

- Understand the difference between leadership and management
- Describe transactional leadership versus transformational leadership
- Define meta-leadership and understand why it is an effective tool for crisis leaders
- Understand why prepared leaders must possess the skills and tools necessary to lead in unfamiliar situations

▶ The Prepared Leader

In many ways, the characteristics of a prepared leader mirror the characteristics of a prepared organization. In the preparedness space, leaders may frequently find themselves in the midst of disaster response operations that are complex and require high-consequence decision-making. Leaders need to have the skills and a readily accessible "toolbox" for effectively managing these disaster responses. Prepared leaders must establish clear lines of coordination and management within their teams and across other agencies and departments, be effective communicators in times of crisis, and push their organizations to constantly learn from emergency responses, both their own and those of others. The American College of Healthcare Executives (ACHE) encourages leaders to continuously undertake the following actions to increase preparedness:

- Maintain a relevant and current emergency/disaster plan
- Focus the plan to address the most likely scenario(s)
- Develop an Incident Command System
- Assess resource availability
- Plan for continuity of operations
- Develop protocols to guarantee appropriate resource distribution/allocation
- Address employee/patient/family safety
- Design appropriate communication/coordination protocols both internally and externally[1]

Each of these items is designed to ensure that organizations and the responders within them are prepared to respond to emergencies when they arise. However, being a *prepared leader* is more complicated than ensuring your organization is prepared to respond to an emergency. Being a prepared leader means that you have acquired the skills to lead, as described above, and also to maintain an analytic mind at all times to learn from past lessons, anticipate the unexpected that is to come, and build collaboration and consensus along the way.

▶ Transactional Versus Transformational Leadership

Two common types of leadership are transactional and transformational. Transactional leaders typically work within an existing organizational culture that generally works well and does not require dramatic change. These leaders tend to focus on supervision, organization, and group performance. Transactional leaders tend to respond to situations rather than encourage change in behavior or results. Traditional performance management tools, such as bonuses, are often utilized by these types of leaders to reward achievements. Often, they motivate staff by appealing to their self-interests. Historical examples of transactional leaders are Joseph McCarthy and Charles de Gaulle.

Transformational leadership is defined by broad, visionary ideas. Transformational leaders tend to focus on implementing new ideas, motivating staff, and encouraging people to put the group's interest ahead of their own. Rewards are more often intrinsic, appealing to ideals or moral values. Simply put, transformational leaders inspire their followers to embrace and invest in the vision the leader has facilitated to be learned among the collaborative.[2,3] Franklin Delano Roosevelt and Martin Luther King, Jr., are two examples of transformational leaders. **TABLE 14-1** compares the leadership styles of transactional and transformational leaders.

TABLE 14-1 Transactional Versus Transformational Leaders	
Transactional Leadership	**Transformational Leadership**
Leaders are aware of the link between the effort and reward	Leaders arouse emotions in their followers, which motivates them to act beyond the framework of what may be described as exchange relations
Leadership is responsive and its basic orientation is dealing with present issues	Leadership is proactive and forms new expectations in followers
Leaders rely on standard forms of inducement, reward, punishment, and sanction to control followers	Leaders are distinguished by their capacity to inspire and provide individualized consideration, intellectual stimulation, and idealized influence to their followers
Leaders motivate followers by setting goals and promising rewards for desired performance	Leaders create learning opportunities for their followers to motivate and stimulate followers to solve problems
Leadership depends on the leader's power to reinforce subordinates for their successful completion of the bargain	Leaders possess good visioning, rhetorical, and management skills, to develop strong emotional bonds with followers
Leaders often use technical knowledge to determine the change process	Leaders search for adaptive solutions to engage hearts and minds in the change process

Reproduced from Kirimi, B., & Minja, D. (2010). Transformational Corporate Leadership. Integrity Publishers Inc.

Transformational leaders focus on utilizing creativity and innovation to achieve the best outcome for the common good.[3] Transformational leadership is defined by four elements or the 4 "I's." First, **Idealized Influence (II)** is where the leader serves as a role model for followers and is admired by his or her team. Next, **Inspirational Motivation (IM)** is the ability to motivate and inspire followers, typically by triggering emotions tied to greater ideas. Third, **Individualized Characterization (IC)** defines the ability to demonstrate genuine concern for feelings and/or needs of followers. Followers who believe their leader is looking out for them and their best interests will typically reciprocate. Finally, **Intellectual Stimulation (IS)** is "the act of challenging followers to be innovative and creative".[4] Constantly challenging followers to higher levels of performance will often lead to better results.[5]

▶ Crisis Leadership

A crisis requires a different type of leadership than managing day-to-day operations. Lives might be at stake and time is precious, but consequential decisions often must be made without access to complete information or in the face of rapid changes. To manage a crisis successfully, a strong leader must be able to make decisions under intense pressure and stress. Crisis leadership also requires people to understand their organization and people, in terms of both capabilities and gaps. Interagency communication can help an organization address these gaps during a crisis, but leaders must understand those gaps well enough to find the right partners to fill them. The following are 10 key characteristics of crisis leadership. Each characteristic serves a different purpose when responding to an emergency:

1. See things for what they are
2. Pay attention to strategy and detail—sees the big picture without getting caught up in details
3. Consider multiple options
4. Are able to be decisive
5. Can collaborate
6. Can listen to unpopular advice
7. Can remain calm, courageous, and positive
8. Can take risk in the face of risk
9. Can make a decision even when lacking information
10. Is prepared to admit mistakes[6]

▶ Meta-Leadership

One of the most effective methodologies available today for assisting crisis leaders with making high-consequence decisions under intense pressure is meta-leadership. Meta-leadership is a leadership framework for "generating widespread and cohesive action that expands the leader's domain of influence and leverage."[7(p2)] It is designed to enable leadership across organizational lines that develop into a shared course of action and a common purpose among seemingly disparate people and entities focused on different work, typically people and entities over which the leader does not have authority.[7] The meta-leadership model, created by a team of leaders and researchers at Harvard University, was "developed after observing and analyzing the actions of leaders in unprecedented crisis situations—post-9/11 and post-Katrina—and in educational settings with more than 500 senior U.S. government leaders".[7] The strength of the framework comes from the forging of strategic connections outside of one's own organization to achieve greater impact, leveraging the skills and resources of many instead of a few. There are three broad dimensions to meta-leadership: the Person, the Situation, and Connectivity. The dimensions are complementary and reinforcing to one another. This interdependence and interconnectedness help ensure success for the leader who uses the framework. A meta-leader utilizes all of the dimensions together, to varying degrees, to maximize their impact. **FIGURE 14-1** displays the three dimensions and how they correspond to one another.

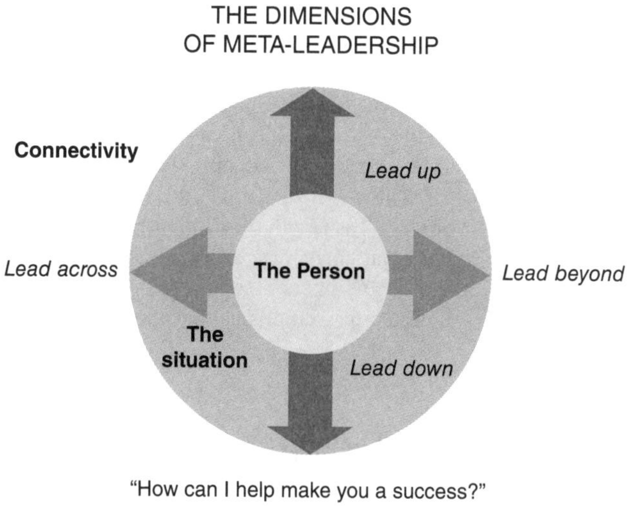

THE DIMENSIONS
OF META-LEADERSHIP

"How can I help make you a success?"

FIGURE 14-1 Dimensions of meta-leadership

Data from Marcus LJ, Dorn BC, Henderson J, McNulty EJ. Meta-Leadership: A Framework for Building Leadership Effectiveness. *A Working Paper*. National Preparedness Leadership Initiative. Cambridge, MA: Harvard School of Public Health; 2015.

The Person

The first dimension of meta-leadership is **the Person**. Meta-leaders must know themselves and "the impact they have on others".[7] Likely the most critical component of leaders knowing themselves is their self-awareness of their own emotional intelligence, how they manage their emotions in high-stress situations. In public health emergencies, leaders must oversee complex, large-scale initiatives and operations. In addition to self-awareness and emotional intelligence, self-regulation, motivation, and the willingness to take on large challenges are additional characteristics that have been shown to correlate with effective leadership. When these characteristics are present in a leader, it is believed that they enable the leader to better understand others.[7]

The Situation

The second dimension of meta-leadership is **the Situation** or environment. During any crisis, there typically is a large degree of ambiguity. Leaders must be able to operate in situations where information changes by the minute and much is unknown, yet somehow to maintain situational awareness and be able to communicate such to others around them. They must be able to display patience and maintain perspective without being consumed by the changing conditions on the ground. These complex and often highly emotional situations are further complicated by the number of stakeholders, including responders and victims, thus making assessment of the situation that much more difficult. Meta-leaders understand that these situations are fluid and can quickly and accurately summarize the situation on the ground, identify the problem, provide context, and quickly disseminate information to all parties involved.

Connectivity

The final dimension of meta-leadership is **Connectivity**. Connectivity speaks to the meta-leader's ability to foster consensus among all those involved and "connect" all participants under a single vision or strategy. Meta-leaders are able to move partners and stakeholders together for an aligned interest, aimed solely at solving the problems at hand, as opposed to any individual, disparate interests or goals. This dimension in particular requires great skill, as it is in this dimension that the meta-leader is exercising the greatest degree of authority over other stakeholders or participants. This "influence beyond your authority" phenomenon is critical to meta-leaders, as it enables them to move persons and organizations out of siloed behavior and to more cohesive operational positions.[7]

▶ Performance Management and Metrics

Large-scale public health emergencies require a sophisticated, coordinated response involving multiple stakeholders across jurisdictions and levels of government in order to protect the public health and minimize casualties. But how does a leader know that the response will be effective and the best use of existing resources to maximize the benefits? Also, when multiple agencies are responding and implementing different strategies, how does a leader know that his or her organization's strategy is the right one?

Performance management is an attempt to quantitatively measure the effectiveness of a response by monitoring actions and results. Performance management can save lives by identifying what practices achieve the best outcomes. To effectively measure overall response, proper metrics must be used and interpreted correctly. A prepared leader is not afraid of the outcomes of performance metrics and the evaluation of capabilities. A prepared leader sees this data as a valuable resource that will aid in identifying any gaps in preparedness planning.

▶ Conclusion

Leadership is a deliberate skill. One must work at developing and refining leadership skills and abilities. Leadership involves the ability to create a vision and convince others to share in that vision. There are multiple leadership styles that can be utilized to motivate others to do their work. The meta-leadership framework enables leaders to manage complex problems with multiple stakeholders to negotiate a shared vision. Meta-leaders align the core interests, motivations, and values of different organizations to develop an integrated vision and set of actions to create change.

Public health emergency preparedness is rapidly changing. Preparedness as a field, including the standards and practices that govern it, changes almost daily. It is difficult to predict where preparedness will be in the future, based on where it is in the present. Leaders, prepared leaders, need to possess the tools and skills to be able and willing to lead in times of discomfort and uncertainty. Public health, emergency preparedness, and the public health infrastructure in general need sound, level-headed thinking in leaders, who have the ability to lead others through a shared vision aimed at achieving the most good for the most people. As this final chapter was being written, Hurricane Harvey was ravaging Houston, Texas, and the Gulf Coast region. From a humanitarian perspective, it was heart-wrenching to see the damage and destruction, as it ripped apart the lives of so many Texans. Many of these same people migrated to the Houston area following Hurricane Katrina in 2005. These two disaster events highlight the need for equity and fairness to be built into emergency plans, as well as the need for leaders to think beyond what is present today. In 2005, we all thought there could never be another Hurricane Katrina–like storm, yet here we are.

Discussion Questions

1. What is the difference between transactional and transformational leadership?
2. Think about the last leadership experience you had. Would you describe your style as transactional or transformational? What was the distinguishing characteristic of your leadership style versus the alternate?
3. What is meta-leadership? Describe the three dimensions of meta-leadership. Explain the value in the interconnectedness of the three dimensions.

References

1. American College of Healthcare Executives. Healthcare executives' role in emergency preparedness. Available at https://www.ache.org/policy/emergency_preparedness.cfm. Revised November 2013. Accessed August 26, 2017.
2. Hartog DN, Muijen JJ, Koopman PL. Transactional versus transformational leadership: an analysis of the MLQ. *J Occup Organ Psychol.* 1997;70(1):19–34.
3. Aarons GA. Transformational and transactional leadership: association with attitudes toward evidence-based practice. *Psychiatric Serv (Washington, DC).* 2006;57(8):1162–1169. doi:10.1176/appi.ps.57.8.1162.
4. Avolio BJ, Waldman DA, Yammarino FJ. Leading in the 1990s: the Four I's of transformational leadership. *J Eur Ind Train.* 1991;15(4). doi:10.1108/03090599110143366.
5. Rowitz, L. *Public Health Leadership: Putting Principles Into Practice.* 2nd ed. Sudbury, MA: Jones and Bartlett Publishers; 2009.
6. Rowe P. Great crisis leaders: 10 key characteristics. Available at https://www.bernsteincrisismanagement.com/newsletter/crisis-manager-081124.html. Published 2008. Accessed August 30, 2017.
7. Marcus LJ, Dorn BC, Henderson J, McNulty EJ. *Meta-Leadership: A Framework for Building Leadership Effectiveness. A Working Paper.* National Preparedness Leadership Initiative. Cambridge, MA: Harvard School of Public Health; 2015.

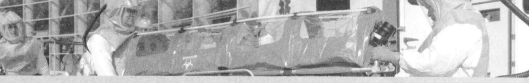

Index